Virtual Clinical Excursions

for

McCance and Huether:

PATHOPHYSIOLOGY:
The Biologic Basis for Disease in Adults and Children
4th Edition

Virtual Clinical Excursions

for

McCance and Huether:
PATHOPHYSIOLOGY:
The Biologic Basis for Disease in Adults and Children
4th Edition

prepared by

Kathy Baldwin, RN, PhD, CEN, CCRN, ANP, GNP
and
Jay Shiro Tashiro, PhD, RN

Virtual Clinical Excursions CD-ROM prepared by

Jay Shiro Tashiro, PhD, RN
Director of Systems Design
Wolfsong Informatics
Sedona, Arizona

Gina Long, RN, DNSc
Assistant Professor, Department of Nursing
College of Health Professions
Northern Arizona University
Flagstaff, Arizona

Ellen Sullins, PhD
Director of Research
Wolfsong Informatics
Sedona, Arizona

Michael Kelly, MS
Director of the Center for Research and
Evaluation of Advanced Technologies
in Education
Northern Arizona University
Flagstaff, Arizona

The development of *Virtual Clinical Excursions* Volume 1 was partially funded by the
National Science Foundation, under grant DUE 9950613.
Principal investigators were Tashiro, Sullins, Long, and Kelly.

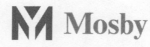

Mosby

A Harcourt Health Sciences Company

St. Louis   London   Philadelphia   Sydney   Toronto

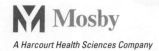

Vice President and Publishing Director, Nursing: Sally Schrefer
Executive Editor: June Thompson
Managing Editor: Michele Trope
Project Manager: Gayle Morris
Designer: Wordbench
Cover Art: Kathi Gosche

NOTICE

Pharmacology is an ever-changing field. Standard safety precautions must be followed, but as new research and clinical experience broaden our knowledge, changes in treatment and drug therapy may become necessary or appropriate. Readers are advised to check the most current product information provided by the manufacturer of each drug to be administered to verify the recommended dose, the method and duration of administration, and contraindications. It is the responsibility of the licensed prescriber, relying on experience and knowledge of the patient, to determine dosages and the best treatment for each individual patient. Neither the publisher nor the editor assumes any liability for any injury and/or damage to persons or property arising from this publication.

Mosby, Inc.
A Harcourt Health Sciences Company
11830 Westline Industrial Drive
St. Louis, Missouri 63146

Printed in the United States of America

International Standard Book Number: 0-323-01733-9

01 02 03 04 05 WB/EB 9 8 7 6 5 4 3 2 1

*Workbook
prepared by*

Kathy Baldwin, RN, PhD, CEN, CCRN, ANP, GNP
Associate Professor of Nursing
Texas Christian University

Jay Shiro Tashiro, PhD, RN
Director of Systems Design
Wolfsong Informatics
Sedona, Arizona

Textbook

Kathryn L. McCance, RN, PhD
Professor, College of Nursing
University of Utah
Salt Lake City, Utah

Sue E. Huether, RN, PhD
Professor, College of Nursing
University of Utah
Salt Lake City, Utah

Contents

Getting Started

GETTING SET UP

■ MINIMUM SYSTEM REQUIREMENTS

Virtual Clinical Excursions is a hybrid CD, so it runs on both Macintosh and Windows platforms. To use *Virtual Clinical Excursions*, you will need one of the following systems:

- **Windows™**

  Windows 2000, 95, 98, NT 4.0
  IBM compatible computer
  Pentium II processor (or equivalent)
  300 MHz
  96 MB
  800 × 600 screen size
  256 color monitor
  100 MB hard drive space
  12× CD-ROM drive
  Soundblaster 16 soundcard compatibility
  Stereo speakers or headphones

- **Macintosh®**

  MAC OS 9.04
  Apple Power PC G3
  300 MHz
  96 MB
  800 × 600 screen size
  256 color monitor
  100 MB hard drive space
  12× CD-ROM drive
  Stereo speakers or headphones

Ideally, the system you use should have at least 200 MB of free disk space on your hard drive. There are commercially available desktop utility programs that can help clean up your hard drive. No other applications besides the operating system should be running at the time *Virtual Clinical Excursions* is running.

■ INSTALLING *VIRTUAL CLINICAL EXCURSIONS*

Virtual Clinical Excursions is designed to run from a set of files on your hard drive and a CD in your CD-ROM. Minimal installation is required.

- **Windows™**

    1. Start Microsoft Windows and insert *Virtual Clinical Excursions* **Disk 1 (Installation)** in the CD-ROM drive.
    2. Click the **Start** icon on the taskbar and select the **Run** option.
    3. Type d:\setup.exe (where "d:\" is your CD-ROM drive) and press OK.
    4. Follow the on-screen instructions for installation.
    5. Remove *Virtual Clinical Excursions* **Disk 1 (Installation)** from your CD-ROM drive.
    6. Restart your computer.

- **Macintosh®**

    1. Insert *Virtual Clinical Excursions* **Disk 1 (Installation)** in the CD-ROM drive. The disk icon will appear on your desktop.
    2. Double-click on the disk icon.
    3. Double-click on the icon **Install Virtual Clinical Excursions**.
    4. Follow the on-screen instructions for installation.
    5. Remove *Virtual Clinical Excursions* **Disk 1 (Installation)** from your CD-ROM drive
    6. Restart your computer.

■ HOW TO RESET YOUR MONITOR TO 256 COLORS

This software will only run if the monitor is set at 256 colors. To reset your monitor:

- **Windows™**

    1. Choose **Settings** from the **Start** menu.
    2. Choose **Control Panel**.
    3. Double-click on the **Display** icon.
    4. Click on the **Settings** tab.
    5. In the **Colors** drop-down menu, click on the arrow to show more settings.
    6. Click on **256 Colors**.
    7. Click on **Apply**.
    8. Click on **OK**.
    9. If the system asks whether you wish to restart your computer to accept these settings, click on **Yes**.

- **Macintosh®**

    1. Choose the **Monitors** control panel.
    2. Change the color display to **256**.

■ **HOW TO USE DISK 2 (PATIENTS' DISK)**

- **Windows™**

  When you want to work with the five patients in the virtual hospital, follow these steps:

  1. Insert *Virtual Clinical Excursions* **Disk 2 (Patients' Disk)** into your CD-ROM drive.
  2. Double-click on the icon **Shortcut to Virtual Clinical Excursions**, which can be found on your desktop. This will load and run the program.

- **Macintosh®**

  When you want to work with the five patients in the virtual hospital, follow these steps:

  1. Insert *Virtual Clinical Excursions* **Disk 2 (Patients' Disk)** into your CD-ROM drive.
  2. Double-click on the icon **Shortcut to Virtual Clinical Excursions**, which can be found on your desktop. This will load and run the program.

■ **QUALITY OF VISUALS, SPEED, AND COMMON PROBLEMS**

Virtual Clinical Excursions uses the Apple QuickTime media layer system. This includes Quick-Time Video and QuickTime VR Video, which allow for high-quality graphics and digital video. The graphics seen in the *Virtual Clinical Excursions* courseware should be of high quality with good color. If the movies and graphics appear blocky or otherwise low-quality, check to see whether your video card is set to "thousands of colors."

Note: Virtual Clinical Excursions is not designed to function at a 256-color depth. (You may need to go to the Control Panel and change the Display settings.) If you don't see any digital video options, please check that QuickTime is installed correctly.

The system should respond quickly and smoothly. In particular, you should not see any jerky motions or unannounced long delays as you move through the virtual hospital settings, interact with patients, or access information resources. If you notice slow, jerky, or delayed software responses, it may mean that your particular system requires additional RAM, your processor does not meet the basic requirements, or your hard drive is full or too fragmented. If the videos appear banded or subject to "breakup," you may need to find an updated video driver for the computer's video card. Please consult the manufacturer of the video card or computer for additional video drivers for your machine.

■ **TECHNICAL SUPPORT**

Technical support for this product is available at no charge by calling the Technical Support Hotline between 9 a.m. and 5 p.m. (Central Time), Monday through Friday. Inside the United States, call 1-800-692-9010. Outside the United States, call 314-872-8370.

A QUICK TOUR

Welcome to *Virtual Clinical Excursions*, a virtual hospital setting in which you can work with five complex patient simulations and also learn to access and evaluate the information resources that are essential for high-quality patient care.

The virtual hospital, Red Rock Canyon Medical Center, is a teaching hospital for Canyonlands State University. Within the medical center, you will work on a medical-surgical floor with a realistic architecture as well as access information resources. The floor plan in which the patient scenarios unfold is constructed from a model of a real medical center. The medical-surgical unit has:

- Five patient rooms (Room 302, Room 303, Room 304, Room 309, Room 310)
- A Nurses' Station (Room 312)
- A Supervisor's Office (Room 301)
- Two conference rooms (Room 307, Room 308)
- A nurses' lounge (Room 306)

■ BEFORE YOU START

Make sure you have your textbook nearby when you use the *Virtual Clinical Excursions Patients' Disk*. You will want to consult topic areas in your textbook frequently while working with the CD and using this workbook.

■ SUPERVISOR'S OFFICE (ROOM 301)

Just like a real-world clinical rotation, you have to let someone know when you arrive on the hospital floor—and you have to let someone know when you leave the floor. This process is completed in the Supervisor's Office (Room 301).

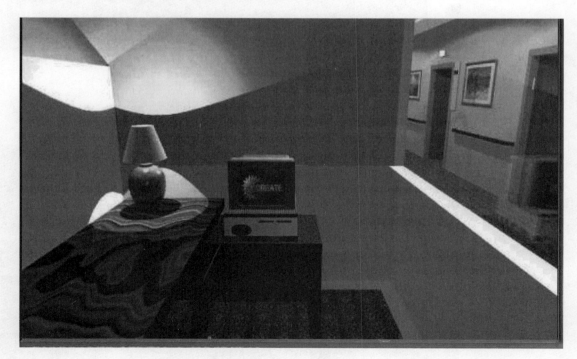

To get a 360° view of where you are "standing":

- Place the cursor in the middle of the screen.
- Hold down the mouse.
- Drag either right or left.

You will see you are in a room with an alcove to your left and a door behind you. To move into the hallway, place the cursor in the door opening and click. Once you are in the hallway, hold down the mouse and make a 360° turn.

In one direction, you will see:

- An exit sign
- An elevator
- A waiting room

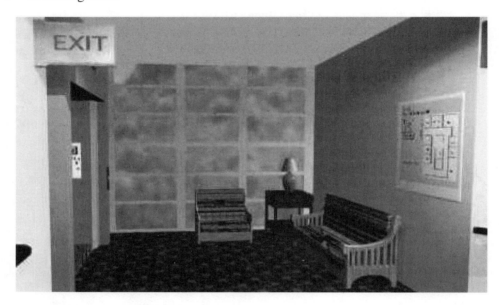

In the other direction, you will see a:

- Patient room
- Mobile computer

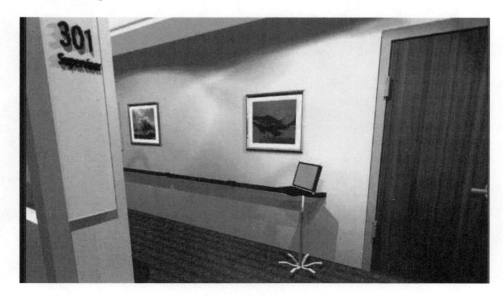

Move the cursor to a new place along the hallway outside the Supervisor's Office and click again. (Always try to place the cursor in the middle of the screen.) You should be moving along the hallway. Remember, at any point you can hold down the mouse and turn 360° in either direction. You can also hold down and move the mouse to the top or bottom of the frame, giving you views looking up or down.

■ READING ROOM

Go back into the Supervisor's Office by clicking on anything inside the room. Explore the Supervisor's Office (Room 301), and you will find another computer. This computer is a link to Canyonlands State University, the simulated university associated with the Red Rock Canyon Medical Center. Double-click on this computer, and a Web browser screen will be launched, which will open the Medical-Nursing Library in Canyonlands State University.

Click on the **Reading Room** icon, and you will see a table of icons that allows you to read short learning modules on a variety of anatomy and physiology topics.

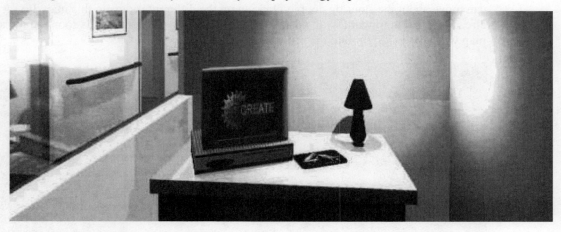

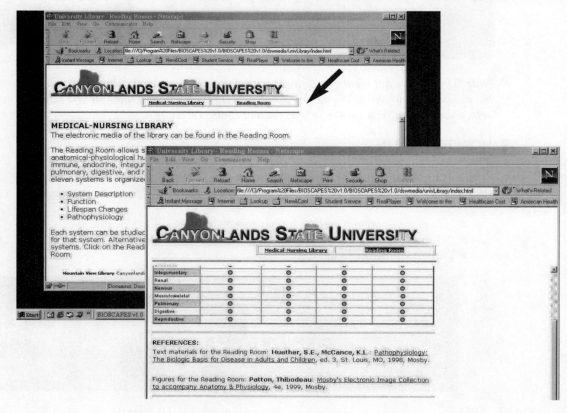

When you are ready to exit the reading room, go to the **File** icon on the browser, look at the drop-down menu, and select **Exit** or **Close**, depending on your Web browser. The browser will close, and once again you will be looking at the computer in the Supervisor's Office.

■ FLOOR MAP AND ANIMATED MAP

Move into the hallway outside the Supervisor's Office and turn right. A floor map can be found on the wall in the waiting area opposite the elevator and exit sign. To get there, click on anything in the waiting area. You should be able to see the map now, but you may not be close enough to open it. Click again on an object in the waiting area; this will move you closer. Turn to the right until you can see the map. Double-click on the map, and you will get a close-up view of the medical-surgical floor's layout. Click on the **Return** icon to exit this close-up view of the floor map.

Compare the floor map on the wall with the animated map in the upper right-hand corner of your screen. The green dot follows your position on the floor to show you where you are. You can move about the floor by double-clicking on the different rooms in this map. If you have already signed in to work with a patient, double-clicking on the patient's room on the animated map will take you right into the room.

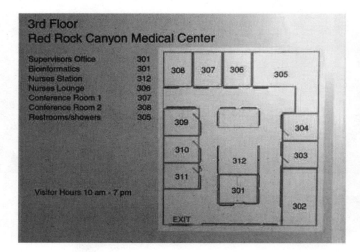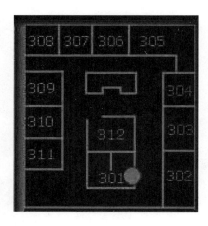

Note: If you have not signed in to work with a patient, double-clicking on a patient's room on the animated map will take you to the hallway right outside the room. If you have not yet selected a patient, you cannot access patient rooms or records.

■ HOW TO SIGN IN

To select a patient, you will need to sign in on the desktop computer in the Supervisor's Office (Room 301). Double-click on the computer screen, and a log-on screen will appear.

- Replace *Student Name* with your name.
- Replace the student ID number with your student ID number.
- Click **Continue** in the lower right side of the screen.

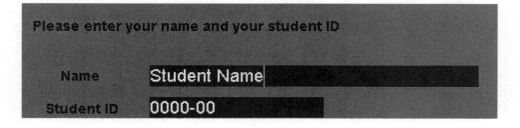

■ HOW TO SELECT A PATIENT

You can choose any one of five patients to work with. For each patient you can select either of two 4-hour shifts on Tuesday or Thursday (0700–1100 or 1100–1500). You can also select a Friday morning period in which you can review all of the data for the patient you selected. You will not, however, be able to visit patients on Friday, only review their records.

■ PATIENT LIST

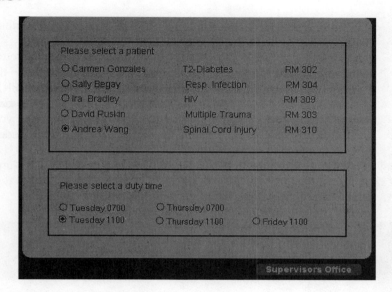

- **Carmen Gonzales (Room 302)**

  Diabetes mellitus, type 2 – An older Hispanic female with an infected leg that has become gangrenous. She has type 2 diabetes mellitus, as well as complications of congestive heart failure and osteomyelitis.

- **David Ruskin (Room 303)**

  Motor vehicle accident – A young adult African-American male admitted with a possible closed head injury and a severely fractured right humerus following a car-bicycle accident. He undergoes an open reduction and internal fixations of the right humerus.

- **Sally Begay (Room 304)**

  Respiratory infection – A Native American woman initially suspected to have a Hantavirus infection. She has a confirmed diagnosis of bacterial lung infection. This patient's complications include chronic obstructive pulmonary disease and inactive tuberculosis.

- **Ira Bradley (Room 309)**

  HIV-AIDS – A Caucasian adult male in late-stage HIV infection admitted for an opportunistic respiratory infection. He has complications of oral fungal infection, malnutrition, and wasting. Patient-family interactions also provide opportunities to explore complex psychosocial problems.

- **Andrea Wang (Room 310)**

  Spinal cord injury – A young Asian female who entered the hospital after a diving accident in which her T6 was crushed, with partial transection of the spinal cord. After a week in ICU, she has been transferred to the Medical-Surgical unit, where she is being closely monitored.

Note: You can select only one patient for one time period. If you are assigned to work with multiple patients, return to the Supervisor's Office to switch from one patient to another.

■ HOW TO FIND A PATIENT'S RECORDS

Nurses' Station (Room 312)

Within the Nurses' Station, you will see:

1. A blue notebook on the counter—this is the Medication Administration Record (MAR).
2. A bookshelf with patient charts.
3. Two desktop computers—the computer to the left of the bulletin board is used to access Red Rock Canyon Medical Center's Intranet; the computer to the right beneath the bookshelf is used to access the Electronic Patient Record (EPR). *(Note: You can also access the EPR from the mobile computer outside the Supervisor's Office, next to Room 302.)*
4. A bulletin board—this contains important information for students.

As you use these resources, you will always be able to return to the Nurses' Station (Room 312) by clicking either a **Nurses' Station** icon or a **3rd Floor** icon located next to the red cross in the lower right-hand corner of the computer screen.

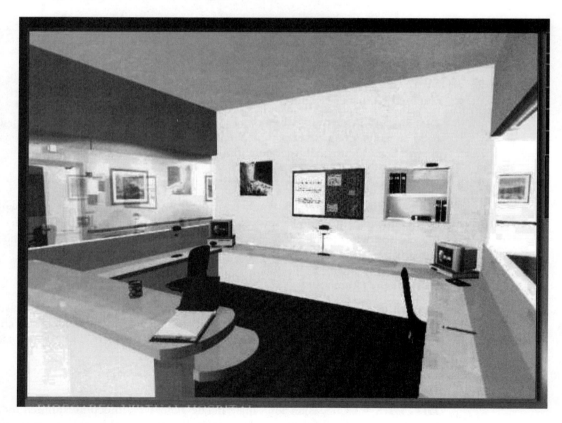

1. Medication Administration Record (MAR)

The blue notebook on the counter in the Nurses' Station (Room 312) is the Medication Administration Record (MAR), listing current 24-hour medications for each patient. Simply click on the MAR, and it opens like a notebook. Tabs allow you to select patients by room number. Each MAR sheet lists the following:

- Medications
- Route and dosage of medications
- Times of administration of medication

The MAR changes each day.

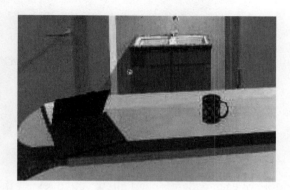

START	END	MEDICATION	2301 0700	0701 1500	1501 2300
		Cefoxitin, 2 g IVPB q6h	~~0300~~ *LG*	~~0900~~ *JS* 1500	2100
		Glyburide, 3.0 mg PO qA.M., with breakfast		~~0800~~ *JS*	
		Blood Glucose, AC and HS 0730 = 260, 1100 = 170		~~0730~~ *JS* ~~1100~~ *JS*	
		Decrease D$_5$ 0.45 NS, 20 cc/hour	~~0600~~ *LG*		
		Morphine Sulfate, IM 2-5 mg q1-2h, PRN for severe pain 5mg @ 0300, 0600 LG 5mg @ 0800	~~0300~~ *LG* ~~0600~~ *LG*	~~0800~~ *JS*	

PATIENT: Gonzales, Carmen   MR# 20194873   DAY: Tuesday

118%   1 of 1   8 x 14 in

302   303   304   309   310

2. Charts

In the back right-hand corner of the Nurses' Station (Room 312) is a bookshelf with patient charts. To open a chart:

- Double-click on the bookshelf.
- Click once on the chart of your choice.

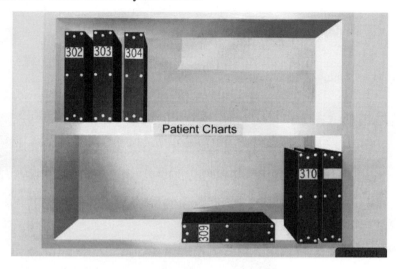

Tabs at the bottom of each patient's chart allow you to review the following data:

- Physical & History*
- Physicians' Notes
- Physicians' Orders
- Nurses' Notes
- Diagnostics Reports

- Expired MARs
- Health Team Reports
- Surgeons' Notes
- Other Reports

"Flip" forward by selecting a tab or backward by clicking on the small chart icon in the lower right side of your screen. (**Flip Back** appears on this icon once you have moved beyond the first tab.) As in the real world, the data in each patient's chart changes daily.

Note: Physical & History is a seven-page PDF file for Carmen Gonzales, David Ruskin, and Ira Bradley. Physical & History is a five-page PDF file for Andrea Wang and Sally Begay. Remember to scroll down to read all pages.

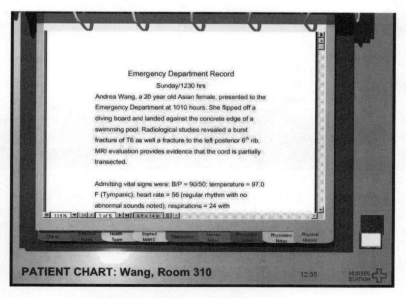

3. Two Computers

◆ **Electronic Patient Record (EPR)**

You can only access an Electronic Patient Record (EPR) once you have signed in and selected the patient in the Supervisor's Office (Room 301). The EPR can be accessed from two computers:

- Desktop computer under the bookshelf in the Nurses' Station (Room 312)
- Mobile computer outside the Supervisor's Office, next to Room 302

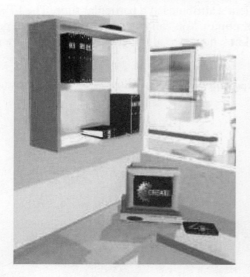 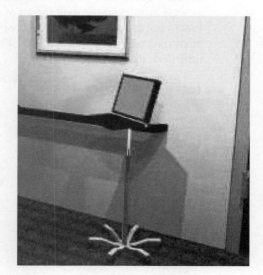

To access a patient's EPR:

- Double-click on the computer screen.
- Type in the password—it will always be **rn2b**.
- Click on **Access Records**.
- Click on the patient's name, then on **Access EPR** (or simply double-click on the patient's name).

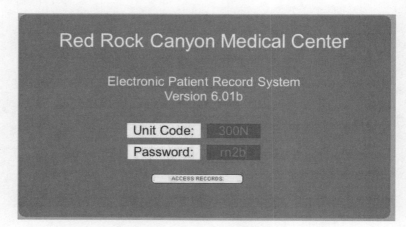

Red Rock Canyon Medical Center

Electronic Patient Record System
Version 6.01b

Unit Code: 300N
Password: rn2b

ACCESS RECORDS

*Note: Do **not** press the Return/Enter key. If you make a mistake, simply delete the password, reenter it, and click **Access Records**. You will then enter the records system, where you find a list of patients.*

The EPR form represents a composite of commercial versions being used in hospitals and clinics. You can access the EPR:

- For a patient
- To review existing data
- To enter data you collect while working with a patient

The EPR is updated daily, so no matter what day or part of a shift you are working, there will be a current EPR with the patient's data from the past days of the current hospital stay. This type of simulated EPR allows you to examine how data for different attributes have changed over time, as well as to examine data for all of a patient's attributes at a particular time. The EPR is fully functional (as it is in a real-life hospital or clinic). You can enter such data as blood pressure, heart rate, and temperature. The EPR will not, however, allow you to enter data for a previous time period.

At the lower left corner of the EPR, there are nine icons that allow you to view different types of patient data:

- Assessment
- Admissions
- Urinanalysis
- Vital Signs
- ADL

- Blood Gases
- I&O
- Chemistry
- Hematology

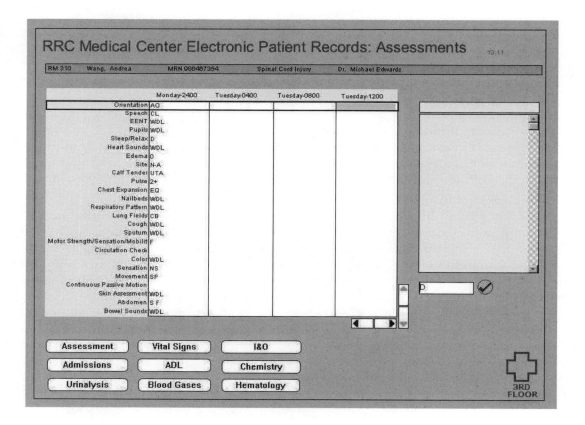

Remember, each hospital or clinic selects its own codes. The codes in the Red Rock Canyon Medical Center may be different from ones you have seen in clinical rotations that have computerized patient records.

You use the codes for the data type, selecting the code to describe your assessment findings and typing that code in the box in the lower right side of the screen, to the left of the checkmark symbol (✓).

Once the data are typed in this box, they are entered into the patient's record by clicking on the checkmark (✓). Make sure you are in the correct cell by looking for the placement of the blue box in the table. That box identifies which cell the database is "looking" at for any given moment.

You can leave the EPR by clicking on the **3rd Floor** icon in the lower right corner. This takes you back into the Nurses' Station (Room 312).

◆ **Intranet**

The computer on the left of the bulletin board in the Nurses' Station (Room 312) is dedicated to Red Rock Canyon Medical Center's **Intranet**. This system contains resources related to working within the hospital. Again, a double click on the screen will activate the computer. A Web browser will come up with four options (Hospital News, Employment, InfoStat, and Home). Navigate within the Intranet just as you would within a Web-based Internet site. Click on **Hospital News** and read some of the articles. The Employment icon opens a screen with descriptions of jobs available in the hospital. The InfoStat icon will connect the hospital Intranet to the Internet. *(Note: This option searches for your Internet connection, activates that connection, and takes you to the publisher's Website for your textbook.)* When in doubt, click on **Home**, which will take you back to the home page for the site.

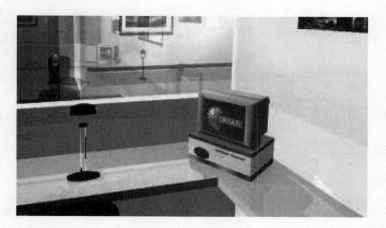

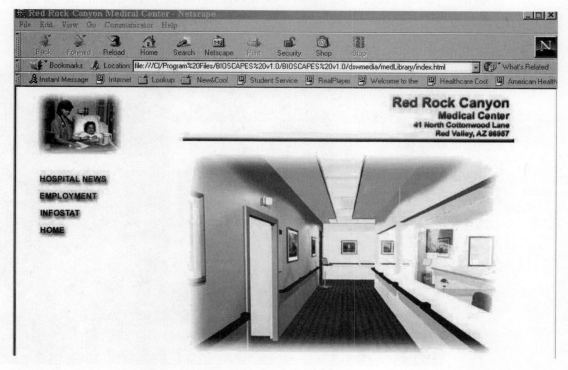

To return to the **Nurses' Station (Room 312)**, exit from the browser. This computer simulates being in a Web environment, so you have to exit from the Intranet by exiting from the browser. Click on **File**, then on **Exit** or **Close** (depending on your browser).

4. Bulletin Board

The bulletin board in the Nurses' Station (Room 312) has important information for students. Click on the board and you can read where reports are being given for patients and where the health team meetings are being held. Lessons in your workbook will direct you to these meetings and reports. Click on **Return** to exit this close-up view of the board.

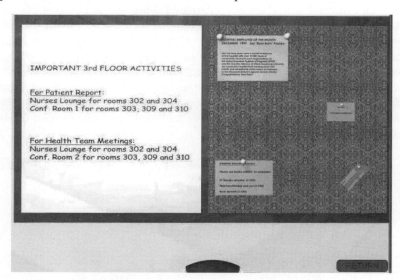

■ VISITING A PATIENT

First, go the Supervisor's Office and sign in to work with Andrea Wang for Tuesday at 0700. Now go to her room. *(Note: The quickest way to get to a patient's room is by double-clicking the room number on the animated map. You can also choose to move through the hallway until you reach the patient's door; then click on the doorknob.)* Once you are inside the room, you will see a still frame of your patient. Below this frame, you will find four icons:

- Vital Signs
- Health History
- Physical
- Medications

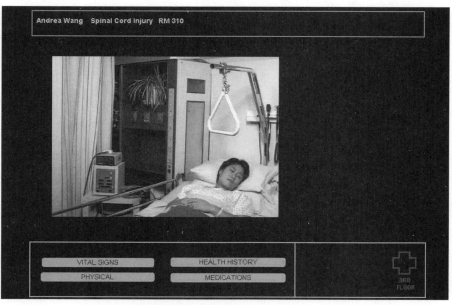

Each of these icons provides the opportunity to assess the patient or the patient's medications. When you click on an icon, you will follow a nurse through the process of collecting assessment data. The nurse will not speak to you but will rely on you to collect the data obtained during patient assessment, to record patient data in the EPR, and sometimes to make decisions after a nurse-patient interaction.

◆ **Vital Signs**

Click on **Vital Signs**; six new icons appear. Each of these new icons allows you to collect data for a particular vital sign. *(Note: You can also see two icons in the right corner.* **Continue Working with Patient** *takes you back to the main menu for this patient. Clicking on* **3rd Floor** *will take you back into the hallway.)* Click on the **Temperature** icon. You will see the nurse take the patient's temperature with a tympanic thermometer. At the end of the measurement, the temperature is shown in the animation of the thermometer to the right of the video screen. These types of interactions allow you to collect data during patient visits.

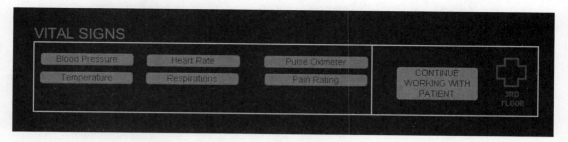

◆ **Physical Examination**

Click **Continue Working with Patient** to return to the main patient menu. Now click the **Physical** icon. Note the different areas of physical examination you can conduct. Try one.

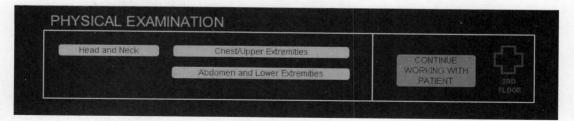

◆ **Health History**

Next, click **Continue Working with Patient** and select the **Health History** icon. In this interactive learning arena, you can ask the patient about her health history. Questions are organized into 12 categories, each of which is accessed by an icon below the video screen. Click on **Culture**, and three new icons appear in the frame to the right of the video. Click on the **Preferred Language** icon, and you will discover the language this patient prefers to use. For each of the 12 question areas, there are three topics you can explore. Thus, there are 36 different question areas related to the health history of each patient.

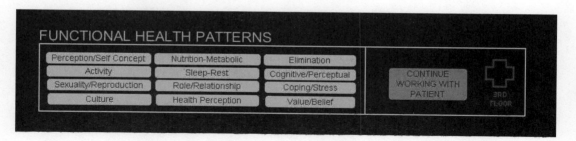

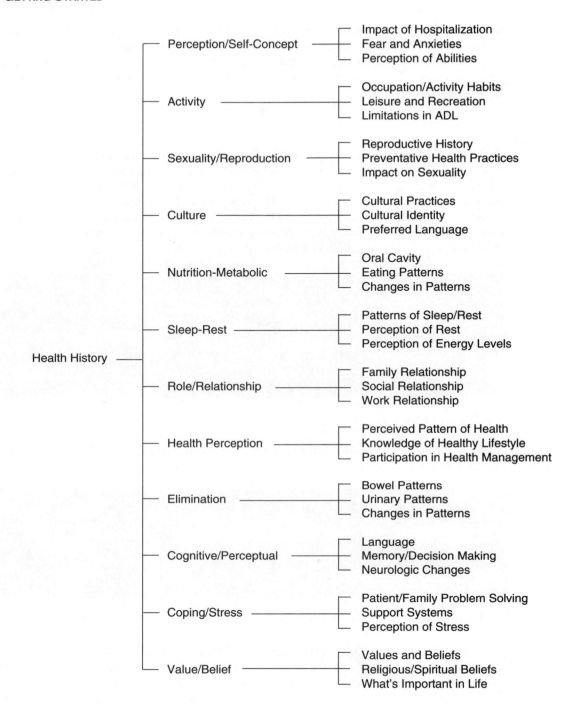

Health History
- Perception/Self-Concept
  - Impact of Hospitalization
  - Fear and Anxieties
  - Perception of Abilities
- Activity
  - Occupation/Activity Habits
  - Leisure and Recreation
  - Limitations in ADL
- Sexuality/Reproduction
  - Reproductive History
  - Preventative Health Practices
  - Impact on Sexuality
- Culture
  - Cultural Practices
  - Cultural Identity
  - Preferred Language
- Nutrition-Metabolic
  - Oral Cavity
  - Eating Patterns
  - Changes in Patterns
- Sleep-Rest
  - Patterns of Sleep/Rest
  - Perception of Rest
  - Perception of Energy Levels
- Role/Relationship
  - Family Relationship
  - Social Relationship
  - Work Relationship
- Health Perception
  - Perceived Pattern of Health
  - Knowledge of Healthy Lifestyle
  - Participation in Health Management
- Elimination
  - Bowel Patterns
  - Urinary Patterns
  - Changes in Patterns
- Cognitive/Perceptual
  - Language
  - Memory/Decision Making
  - Neurologic Changes
- Coping/Stress
  - Patient/Family Problem Solving
  - Support Systems
  - Perception of Stress
- Value/Belief
  - Values and Beliefs
  - Religious/Spiritual Beliefs
  - What's Important in Life

◆ **Medications**

Click **Continue Working with Patient**, and then click the **Medications** icon. Notice that you have three options within this learning environment: Review Medications, Administer, and Hold Medications. Don't click on these now, because you will need to look at this patient's records before you decide whether or not to give medications.

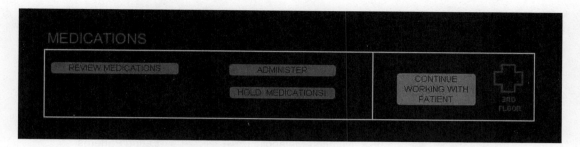

■ HOW TO QUIT OR CHANGE PATIENTS

How to Quit: If necessary, click either the **3rd Floor** icon or the **Nurses' Station** icon (depending on which screen you are currently using) to return to the medical-surgical floor. Then click on the **Quit** icon in the lower right corner of your screen.

How to Change Patients or Shifts: Go to the Supervisor's Office and double-click on the sign-in computer. Click the **Reset** icon. When the next screen appears, select a new patient or a different shift with the same patient.

A DETAILED TOUR

If you wish to understand the capabilities of the virtual hospital, take a detailed tour by going through the following section.

■ WORKING WITH A PATIENT

Sign in and select Carmen Gonzales as your patient for Tuesday at 0700 hours.

To become more familiar with the *Virtual Clinical Excursions Patients' Disk,* try the following exercises. These activities are designed to introduce you to all of the different components and learning opportunities available within the software. Each exercise will ask you to collect data on a patient.

■ REPORT

In hospitals, when one nurse's shift ends and another begins, the outgoing nurse who attended a patient will give a verbal and sometimes a written summary of that patient's condition to the incoming nurse who will assume care for the patient. This summary is called a *report* and is an important source of data to provide an overview of a patient.

Your first task is to get the report on Carmen Gonzales. Go to the bulletin board in the Nurses' Station. Double-click on the board and check the location where the attending nurse from the previous shift will give you report on this patient. Remember, Carmen Gonzales is in Room 302, so look for that room number on the bulletin board. You will find that the report is being given in the Nurses' Lounge (Room 306). Click **Return** to leave this close-up view of the bulletin board. *(Note: You can also find out where reports are being given by moving your cursor across the animated map.)* Go to Room 306 by double-clicking on the animated map. Once inside the room, click on **Report** and then on **Gonzales**. Listen to report and make a list of this patient's problems and high-priority concerns. When you are finished, click on the **3rd Floor** icon to return to the Nurses' Station.

Problems/Concerns

■ **CHARTS**

Find the patient charts in the bookshelf to the right of the bulletin board. Double-click on the bookshelf and find Carmen Gonzales' chart (the one labeled **302**). Click on her chart and read the section called Physical & History, including the Emergency Department Record. Determine from this information why Carmen Gonzales has been admitted to the hospital. In the space below, write a brief summary of why this patient was admitted.

■ **MEDICATIONS**

Open the Medication Administration Record (MAR) by clicking on the blue notebook on the counter of the Nurses' Station. Find the list of medications prescribed for Carmen Gonzales, and write down the medications that need to be given during the time period 0730–0930. For each medication, note dosage, route, and time in the chart below.

Time	Medication	Dosage	Route

Close the MAR and go inside Carmen Gonzales' room (302). Click on the **Medications** icon. You will be responsible for administering the medications ordered during the time period 0730–0930.

To become familiar with the medication options, look at the frame below the video screen. There you will find three opportunities:

- Review Medications
- Administer
- Hold Medications

Click on **Review Medications**. This brings up a frame to the right of the video screen with a list of the medications ordered for the period 0730–0930 hours. Decide whether these medications match what appears within the **Medication Administration Record (MAR)** for this time period. If they do match, you can click the **Administer** icon. If they do not match, you should select **Hold Medications**. When you are finished, click **Continue Working With Patient** to return to the patient care menu.

■ VITAL SIGNS

Vital signs are often considered the traditional signs of life and include body temperature, heart rate, respiratory rate, blood pressure, oxygen saturation of the blood, and the patient's experience of pain.

Inside Carmen Gonzales' room, click on the **Vital Signs** icon. This icon activates a pathway that allows you to measure the patient's vital signs. When you enter this pathway, you will see a short video in which the nurse informs the patient what is about to happen. Six vital signs options appear at the bottom of the screen. Each icon activates a video clip in which the respective vital sign is measured. Relevant vital signs data become available in these videos. For example, click on **Heart Rate**, and a video clip and animation of a radial pulse appear. You can measure the heart rate by counting the animated pulses during a prescribed time.

Try each of the different vital signs options to see what kinds of data are obtained. The vital signs data change over time to reflect the temporal changes you would find in a patient similar to Carmen Gonzales. You will see this most clearly if you "leave" the Tuesday time period you are currently within and "come back" on Thursday. However, you will also find changes throughout any given day (for example, differences between the 0700–1100 and 1100–1500 shifts).

Collect vital signs data for Carmen Gonzales and enter them into the following table. Note the time at which you collected these data.

Vital Signs	Findings/Time
Blood Pressure	
O$_2$ Saturation	
Heart Rate	
Respiratory Rate	
Temperature	
Pain Rating	

After you are done, click on the **3rd Floor** icon in the lower right portion of your screen. This will take you back into the hallway. Move along the hallway (or use the animated map in the upper right corner of your screen) to return to the Nurses' Station. Enter the station, and click on the computer that accesses the Electronic Patient Record (EPR). First you will see the Electronic Patient Record System entry screen. Type in **rn2b** for the password (remember, do *not* press the Return/Enter key). Then click **Access Records**, and you will see a new screen with patients listed. Click on **Carmen Gonzales** and then on **Access EPR**. Now you are in the EPR system. Click on **Vital Signs**, which will open the screen with vital signs data. Use the blue and orange arrows in the lower right-hand corner of the data table to move around within the database. Look at the data collected earlier for each of the vital signs you measured. Use these data to establish a baseline for each of the vital signs.

a. Are any of the data you collected significantly different from the baselines for those vital signs?	Circle One: Yes No
b. If "Yes," which data are different?	

■ PHYSICAL ASSESSMENT

After examining the EPR for vital signs, click the **Assessment** icon and review Carmen Gonzales' data in this area. Once you have reviewed the data and noted any areas of concern to you, close the EPR, enter Carmen Gonzales' room, and click on the **Physical** icon. This will activate the following three options for conducting a physical assessment of the patient:

- Head and Neck
- Chest/Upper Extremities
- Abdomen and Lower Extremities

Click on the **Head and Neck** icon. You will see the nurse conduct an assessment of the head and neck. At the end of the video, a series of icons appear in a frame to the right of the video screen. These icons list the different areas of the head and neck that were examined and the data obtained during the examination. The icons allow you to replay that section of the video in which the particular area was examined.

For example, if you click on **Oculomotor** (the finding is "Oculomotor function intact"), you will see a replay of the assessment of oculomotor function. Each of the icons activates only that portion of the head and neck assessment focused on the particular area described by the icon. The intention is to help you correlate each part of a physical assessment with the data obtained from that assessment—and to give you the opportunity to have the whole assessment of a region conducted beginning to end so that you can learn the process as well as its component parts. Click **Continue Working with Patient** and explore the Chest/Upper Extremities and the Abdomen and Lower Extremities options. For each area, browse through the icons that provide data on a particular area of the assessment. (*Note: The data for certain attributes found during physical assessments change for some patients as you follow them through the virtual week.*)

Focus on the examination of the abdomen and lower extremities by clicking on the option. Pay close attention to the leg wound. In the following table, record the data collected by the nurse during the examination.

Area of Examination	Findings
Abdomen	
Legs	

After you have completed the physical examination of the abdomen and lower extremities, click **Continue Working with Patient** to return to the patient care menu. From there, click on the **3rd Floor** icon and return to the Nurses' Station. Enter the data you collected in Carmen Gonzales' EPR. Compare the data that were already in the record with the data you just collected.

a. Are any of the data you collected significantly different from the baselines for those vital signs?	Circle One: Yes No
b. If "Yes," which data are different?	

■ HEALTH HISTORY

Conduct part of a health history of Carmen Gonzales. Return to her room and click on the **Health History** icon. Twelve health history areas become visible as icons below the video screen. For example, you can see Perception/Self-Concept, Activity, Sexuality/Reproduction, and so on. Note that this patient speaks Spanish and that the nurse has brought in a translator. All of the health history conversations with Carmen Gonzales are completed through translation. Clicking on any of the 12 health history icons reveals three question areas for that category. For example, if you click **Perception/Self-Concept**, a box appears to the right of the video screen with three question areas:

- Impact of Hospitalization
- Fear and Anxieties
- Perception of Abilities

Each of these three areas can be activated by clicking on their respective icons. When an icon is clicked, you will see a video in which your preceptor asks a question in the respective area and the patient answers through the translator.

Since there are 12 health history areas, with three areas of questioning for each, you have access to a total of 36 video clips that provide an opportunity to learn quite a bit about Carmen Gonzales. The questions and responses were chosen for reasons. In fact, conducting an actual health history would not unfold in such discrete and isolated moments; in the real world you would need to follow up some responses with additional questions. Other lessons in this workbook will encourage you to look at each of the health history areas and decide what additional questions need to be asked.

Unlike the vital signs and physical examination findings, the health history data do not change. The developers of *Virtual Clinical Excursions* realized that the number of videos (and the space required for storage) would become too large for the type of educational package we envisioned. We therefore decided to produce only one set of health history data-collecting opportunities. In truth, the health history would probably not change much over a week. Lessons in your workbook may have you collect health history data on the first day of care, or some of the health history queries may be assigned for Tuesday and the others for Thursday.

We recommend that you explore the health history of Carmen Gonzales by choosing some of the 12 categories and asking one or two of the three questions available for each area. When you are done exploring the health history options, leave the patient's room and go to one of the computers that allow you to access the EPR. Browse through the different data fields to see where you would enter data from the health history questions.

Remember: When you are ready to stop working with your *Virtual Clinical Excursions Patients' Disk*, click on the **Quit** icon found in the lower right-hand corner of any of the 3rd floor screens.

■ COLLECTING AND EVALUATING DATA

Each of the patient care activities generates a great deal of assessment data. Remember that after you collect data, you can go to the Nurses' Station or the mobile computer outside Room 302 and enter the data into the EPR. You also can review the data in the EPR, as well as review a patient's chart and MAR. You will get plenty of practice collecting and then evaluating data in the context of the patient's course during previous shifts.

Now, here's an important question for you:

> Did the previous sequence of exercises provide the most efficient way to assess Carmen Gonzales?

For example, you went to the patient's room to get vital signs, then back to the EPR to enter data and compare your finding with extant data. Then, you went back to the patient's room to do a physical examination, and again back to the EPR to enter and review data. If this back-and-forth process of data collection and recording seemed inefficient, remember the following:

- You want to plan all of your nursing activities to maximize efficiency while at the same time optimizing quality of patient care.
- You collect a tremendous amount of data when you work with a patient. Very few people can accurately remember all these data for more than a few minutes. Develop efficient assessment skills, and enter assessment data as soon as possible after collecting them.
- Assessment data are only the starting point for the nursing process.

Make a clear distinction between these first exercises and how you actually provide nursing care. These initial exercises were designed to involve you actively in the use of different software components. This workbook focuses on sensible practices for implementing the nursing process in ways that ensure the highest quality care of patients.

Most importantly, remember that a human being changes through time—and that these changes include both the physical and psychosocial facets of a person as a living organism. Think about this for a moment. Some patients may change physically in a very short time (a patient with emerging myocardial infarction) or more slowly (a patient with chronic illness). Patients' overall physical and psychosocial conditions may improve or deteriorate. They may have effective coping skills and familial support or feel they are alone and full of despair. In fact, each individual is a complex mix of physical and psychosocial elements, and at least some of these elements usually change through time.

Thus it is crucial *not* to think of the nursing process as a simple one-time, five-step procedure:

- Assessment
- Nursing Diagnosis
- Planning
- Implementation
- Evaluation

Rather, it is a creative and systematic approach to delivering nursing care. Furthermore, because all living organisms are constantly changing, we must apply the nursing process over and over. Each time we follow the nursing process for an individual patient, we refine our understanding of that patient's physical and psychosocial conditions based on collection and analyses of many different types of data. *Virtual Clinical Excursions* will help you develop both the creativity and the systematic approach needed to become a nurse who can deliver the highest quality care to all patients.

The following icons are used throughout the workbook to help you quickly identify particular activities and assignments:

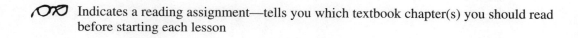 Indicates a reading assignment—tells you which textbook chapter(s) you should read before starting each lesson

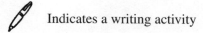 Indicates a writing activity

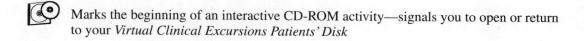 Marks the beginning of an interactive CD-ROM activity—signals you to open or return to your *Virtual Clinical Excursions Patients' Disk*

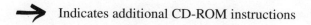 Indicates additional CD-ROM instructions

Indicates questions and activities that require you to consult your textbook

LESSON **1** _____

Cellular Biology

_____

/OꝊ **Reading Assignment:** Cellular Biology (Chapter 1)
Patients: Carmen Gonzales, Room 302
David Ruskin, Room 303
Sally Begay, Room 304
Ira Bradley, Room 309
Andrea Wang, Room 310

Before You Start

In these exercises, you will explore the cellular biology of pathophysiologic conditions in five patients. Before you start, read Chapter 1 in your textbook. (Feel free, however, to review the questions in this lesson first. This may help to focus your reading.) Keep your textbook nearby so that you can consult it frequently as you use the *Virtual Clinical Excursions Patients' Disk* and this workbook.

1. Chapter 1 includes a discussion of eight cellular functions. List and describe these seven functions below.

Cellular Function	**Description**
a.	
b.	

c.

d.

e.

f.

g.

h.

Now apply what you know about these cellular functions to each of the five patients in Red Rock Canyon Medical Center. Before you begin this CD activity, read questions 2 through 11. This will help you focus your review of the data you access. For each patient, sign in for the Tuesday 0700 shift on the desktop computer in the Supervisor's Office. *(Note: You can only sign in for one patient at a time. When you have finished the following steps for the first patient, return to the Supervisor's Office and click on **Reset** to select a new patient. You may work with the patients in any order you choose.)* After you have signed in, go to one of the computers that allow you to access the Electronic Patient Record (EPR)—either the desktop computer under the bookshelf in the Nurses' Station or the mobile computer in the hallway next to Room 302. Click on the computer screen, enter the password (**rn2b**), and click **Access Records**. When the next screen appears, select the patient's name and click on **Access EPR** (or simply double-click on the patient's name). Next, click on **Admissions** and review the Admissions Profile. Now close the EPR and find the patient's chart on the bookshelf in the Nurses' Station. Open the chart and read the Physical & History, paying special attention to the patient's diagnosis. (Remember to scroll down to read all pages.) Once you have completed the previous steps for all five patients, answer the following questions.

2. Based on each patient's diagnosis and history and your understanding of cellular functions, which cellular functions are likely to be altered in each of the five patients? Use the space below to record notes on possible alterations in cellular function for each patient.

Patient	Alterations in Cellular Function

3. From reading the Admissions Profile and the Physical & History for each patient, you should be able to determine that three patients have infections. Who are they?

 4. Explain the role of cellular receptors in infection. (Consult your textbook if necessary.)

5. Which patients will need adequate cellular nutrition?

6. Describe the three phases of food catabolism used to supply cellular energy.

7. Discuss the processes of cellular intake and output of nutrients.

8. Once again, consider what you have learned from each patient's Admissions Profile and Physical & History. Which patients have fractures?

9. Which patients have wounds?

10. For fractures and wounds to heal, new cells must be produced. Using your textbook as a guide, explain the process of cellular reproduction.

11. Which patient has the greatest nutritional need? What data from the chart support your answer?

Altered Cellular and Tissue Biology

 Reading Assignment: Altered Cellular and Tissue Biology (Chapter 2)
Patients: Carmen Gonzales, Room 302
David Ruskin, Room 303
Sally Begay, Room 304
Ira Bradley, Room 309
Andrea Wang, Room 310

Before You Start

You have read about normal cell functioning. Now we turn to altered cellular and tissue biology. Before you start the following exercises, read Chapter 2 in your textbook. Again, make sure you have your textbook nearby when you use the *Virtual Clinical Excursions* CD.

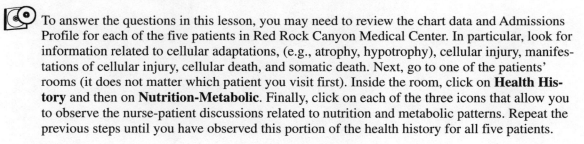 To answer the questions in this lesson, you may need to review the chart data and Admissions Profile for each of the five patients in Red Rock Canyon Medical Center. In particular, look for information related to cellular adaptations, (e.g., atrophy, hypotrophy), cellular injury, manifestations of cellular injury, cellular death, and somatic death. Next, go to one of the patients' rooms (it does not matter which patient you visit first). Inside the room, click on **Health History** and then on **Nutrition-Metabolic**. Finally, click on each of the three icons that allow you to observe the nurse-patient discussions related to nutrition and metabolic patterns. Repeat the previous steps until you have observed this portion of the health history for all five patients.

1. Based on your review of the health history of all five patients, which of them is at greatest risk for atrophy? Explain why.

2. Using Chapter 2 in your textbook as a guide, describe the process of muscular atrophy.

3. Once again, consider your review of the five patients' health histories. Which patients have experienced hypertrophy of their heart muscle because of coronary artery disease?

4. Based on your textbook reading, describe the process of hypertrophy.

5. The five patients have suffered a variety of types of cellular injury. Describe the type of cellular injury found in Carmen Gonzales and Sally Begay as a result of arteriosclerosis from coronary artery disease.

6. Explain the mechanism of the injury you identified in question 5. (Consult Chapter 2 in your textbook if you need help.)

Once again, review the Physical & History section of two of the patient's charts—Sally Begay and Carmen Gonzales.

7. What significant medical history in either patient supports the occurrence of hypoxic cellular injury?

8. Go back through the notes you took on each patient's health history. In particular, review what each patient told the nurse when asked about nutrition and metabolic patterns. Which patient is malnourished?

9. From your reading of textbook Chapters 1 and 2, discuss the effects of nutritional deficits on cellular functioning.

10. Based on your understanding of Ira Bradley's condition, what types of nutritional deficits might result from his disease and his difficulty eating and drinking?

11. From your review of the Admissions Profiles, you should have noted the ethnicity of each patient. Now think about different types of cellular injury and consider the risk for skin cancer related to exposure to sunlight. Which patients have the least risk for skin cancer based on their ethnicity? Why is their risk lower?

12. Discuss the protective effects of melanin on David Ruskin's skin.

 13. Chapter 2 in your textbook describes processes of cellular death. From your review of each patient's chart, you know that one of the patients has an area of necrotic tissue resulting from gangrene. Which patient entered the hospital with gangrene? Where was the infection located?

14. Using the textbook as your guide, describe the processes of necrosis and gangrene.

15. In question 13, you identified a patient with gangrene. What type of gangrene does this patient have?

The Cellular Environment: Fluids and Electrolytes, Acids and Bases

Reading Assignment: The Cellular Environment: Fluids and Electrolytes, Acids and Bases (Chapter 3)

Patients: Carmen Gonzales, Room 302
David Ruskin, Room 303
Sally Begay, Room 304
Ira Bradley, Room 309
Andrea Wang, Room 310

Before You Start

The cells of the body live in a complex environment, and changes in this environment can lead to a variety of problems. Before you start the following exercises, read Chapter 3 in your textbook, although you may want to review the questions first to focus your reading.

In the Supervisor's Office, sign in to work with David Ruskin on Tuesday at 1100. Go into his room and conduct a physical examination by clicking on the **Physical** icon. This will activate three opportunities for performing a physical assessment of the patient. As in all of the patient care pathways, the first scene shows the nurse explaining to the patient what is about to happen. The options for physical assessment include examinations of three different body areas. Click on **Chest/Upper Extremities** and observe as the nurse conducts an assessment of these areas of the body. At the end of the examination, a set of icons appears in a frame to the right of the computer screen listing the areas of the chest and upper extremities that were examined. Clicking on any of these icons allows you to replay that particular section of the examination.

1. What data from the physical examination suggest there has been a fluid disturbance at David Ruskin's fracture site?

2. Explain the pathophysiology of this disturbance. (Consult your textbook if necessary.)

Return to the Supervisor's Office and sign in to work with Sally Begay for the Tuesday 0700 shift. (Remember: You will need to click **Reset** on the sign-in screen to switch patients.) Now go to one of the computers that allow you to access the EPR. Open Sally Begay's EPR and click on **Chemistry**.

3. What was Sally Begay's serum potassium level on Sunday at 0800? What is the normal serum potassium level? What problem might be caused by this patient's serum potassium level?

4. Explain how the diuretic (hydrochlorothiazide) that Sally Begay is taking can cause the problem you identified in question 3.

5. What can the patient do to prevent this problem?

→ Once again, return to the Supervisor's Office; this time, sign in to work with Ira Bradley on Tuesday at 0700. Go to the Nurses' Station, open this patient's chart and review his Physical & History (Remember to scroll down to read all pages.) Now close Ira Bradley's chart and access his EPR. Review the data related to his vital signs and blood chemistry.

6. Was Ira Bradley's serum potassium level elevated on Sunday night? What is the medical term for this condition?

7. What are the most common manifestations of the condition you identified in question 6? Based on your review of Ira Bradley's Physical & History, list findings that could be caused by this condition.

8. What is the normal serum sodium level? (Consult your textbook if necessary.)

9. Was Ira Bradley's serum sodium level elevated on Sunday night? What is the medical term for this condition?

10. What are the most common causes of the condition you identified in question 9? Based on the information in Ira Bradley's EPR and Physical & History, what could be contributing to this condition?

11. In the physiology of humans, age can have an effect on the distribution of body fluids. As an example, consider Carmen Gonzales, who is 56 years old. Explain how her increasing age could affect the distribution of her body fluids.

12. Acid-base disturbances can be caused by a variety of physiologic changes. Think about Andrea Wang. If she develops spinal shock following her spinal cord injury, she is at risk for respiratory depression. What acid-base disturbance results from respiratory depression?

13. Describe the pathophysiology of the disturbance you identified in question 12.

LESSON 4 ———————————————————

Genes, Environment, and Common Diseases

———————————————————————————————————————

Reading Assignment: Genes, Environment, and Common Diseases (Chapter 5)
Patients: Carmen Gonzales, Room 302
   David Ruskin, Room 303
   Sally Begay, Room 304
   Ira Bradley, Room 309
   Andrea Wang, Room 310

Before You Start

Many diseases result from complex interactions among genetic and environmental factors. Read Chapter 5 in your textbook before you start the following exercises and keep the textbook nearby so that you can consult it as you complete this lesson.

In the Supervisor's Office, sign in to work with Carmen Gonzales for the Tuesday 0700 shift. Go to the Nurses' Station, open her chart, and read the Physical & History. (Remember to scroll down to read all pages.) Now repeat the previous steps for each of the patients in Red Rock Canyon Medical Center.

1. Based on your review of the Physical & History for all five patients, identify which of the patients have multifactorial disorders. Below and on the next page, list these patients and the multifactorial disorder each patient suffers. Next, list the general risk factors for each disorder. Finally, identify which of these risk factors each patient has.

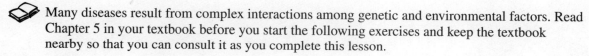

Patient	Disorder	General Risk Factors	Patient's Risk Factors

Patient	Disorder	General Risk Factors	Patient's Risk Factors

➡ Now consider the height and weight of each patient. If necessary, return to each patient's chart and review the Physical & History to find this information. (Remember: You can only sign in for one patient at a time. To check more than one patient's chart, you must return to the Supervisor's Office and select a new patient.)

2. Based on your review of the data, which patient is mildly obese?

3. Obesity is a risk factor for which diseases?

→ Next, review the Family History section of each patient's Physical & History. Also, visit each patient's room and conduct a health history. Focus specifically on the Health Perception category. (Click first on **Health History**, then on **Health Perception**, and listen to the patient's response to each of the three question areas.)

4. Based on your review of all five charts and on the patients' discussion of their own health perception, list below the multifactorial diseases each patient is at risk for developing or has already developed.

Patient	At Risk For	Has Already Developed

LESSON **5** _____

Immunity

_____

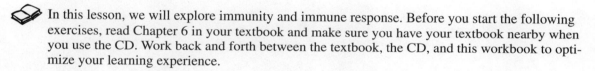 **Reading Assignment:** Immunity (Chapter 6)
Patients: Carmen Gonzales, Room 302
Ira Bradley, Room 309

Before You Start

In this lesson, we will explore immunity and immune response. Before you start the following exercises, read Chapter 6 in your textbook and make sure you have your textbook nearby when you use the CD. Work back and forth between the textbook, the CD, and this workbook to optimize your learning experience.

1. Using your textbook as a guide, describe the characteristics of a normal immune response.

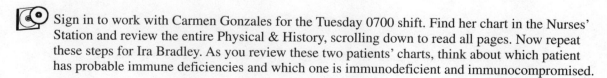 Sign in to work with Carmen Gonzales for the Tuesday 0700 shift. Find her chart in the Nurses' Station and review the entire Physical & History, scrolling down to read all pages. Now repeat these steps for Ira Bradley. As you review these two patients' charts, think about which patient has probable immune deficiencies and which one is immunodeficient and immunocompromised.

2. Which patient—Carmen Gonzales or Ira Bradley—has probable immune deficiencies?

3. What information in the Physical & History section points to probable immune deficiencies for this patient?

4. Carmen Gonzales is 56 years old. What effects will aging have on her immune function?

5. Which patient—Carmen Gonzales or Ira Bradley—is immunodeficient and immunocompromised?

6. According to Chapter 6 in your textbook, what is the primary immunocyte in the immune response?

7. If this immunocyte travels through lymphoid tissue, what type does it become?

8. If this immunocyte travels through the thymus, what type does it become?

9. From your review of the chart data, which patient has AIDS?

10. AIDS affects T cell development, which affects the cell-mediated response. What are the major effects of the cell-mediated immune response?

→ Once again, open Ira Bradley's chart. If necessary, return to the Supervisor's Office and sign in to work with him on Tuesday at 0700.

11. What findings in Ira Bradley's Physical & History are consequences of a severely decreased immunity?

LESSON 6

Inflammation

 Reading Assignment: Inflammation (Chapter 7)
Patients: Carmen Gonzales, Room 302
David Ruskin, Room 303
Sally Begay, Room 304
Ira Bradley, Room 309
Andrea Wang, Room 310

Before You Start

Before you start this lesson, please read Chapter 7 in your textbook. Remember to optimize your learning experience by using the textbook, the CD, and this workbook as complementary resources.

After reading Chapter 7, you know that inflammation is a biochemical and cellular response that can occur in any vascularized tissue. Apply this knowledge as you review the charts of the five patients at Red Rock Canyon Medical Center. For each patient, sign in for the Friday 1100 shift. (The Friday records include all data on the patients from their first day of hospitalization.) After signing in, go to the Nurses' Station and open the patient's chart. Read the Physical & History, looking for evidence of inflammatory response. (Remember to scroll down to read all pages.) Close the chart and access the patient's EPR on the computer under the bookshelf. Review the hematology data, again watching for evidence of inflammatory response.

1. Which patients have developed an acute inflammatory response? For each patient, identify the cause of the response.

2. Using your textbook as a guide and considering what you learned from the patients' charts and EPR data, describe what happens in an acute inflammatory response.

3. Your textbook describes three key plasma protein systems that mediate inflammation. What are these systems?

4. Again using your textbook, name the two main classes of leukocytes that carry out the inflammatory response.

 5. In Chapter 7 of your textbook, review the section that describes systemic inflammatory response. Now evaluate the patient data you have gathered. Which of the five patients should exhibit a systemic inflammatory response?

6. The normal percentage of monocytes (monos) in a white blood cell count is 3%. From your review of the hematology data in the EPR, list the monocyte counts for each of the patients you identified in question 5. Evaluate what each patient's count means.

 7. Your textbook describes the systemic manifestations of acute inflammation. What are the three primary systemic changes?

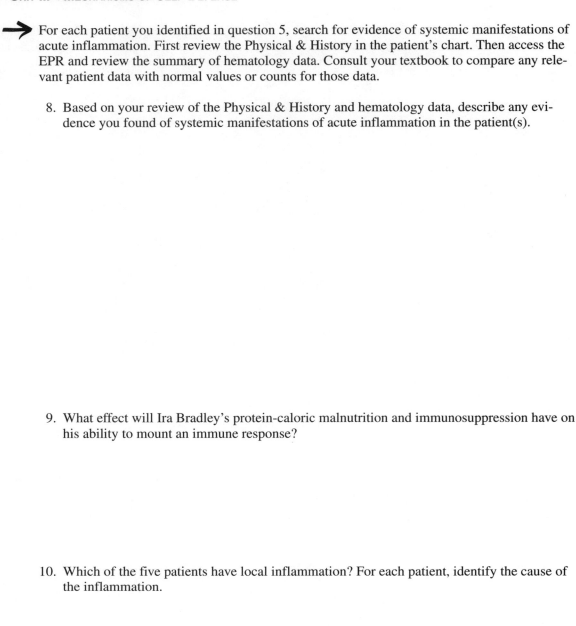 For each patient you identified in question 5, search for evidence of systemic manifestations of acute inflammation. First review the Physical & History in the patient's chart. Then access the EPR and review the summary of hematology data. Consult your textbook to compare any relevant patient data with normal values or counts for those data.

8. Based on your review of the Physical & History and hematology data, describe any evidence you found of systemic manifestations of acute inflammation in the patient(s).

9. What effect will Ira Bradley's protein-caloric malnutrition and immunosuppression have on his ability to mount an immune response?

10. Which of the five patients have local inflammation? For each patient, identify the cause of the inflammation.

11. What are the local manifestations of inflammation?

12. For each patient you identified in question 10, return to the chart and list the local manifestations of inflammation documented in the Physical & History.

13. Which patient is at risk for keloid formation because of his or her ethnicity?

14. Describe the pathophysiology of keloid formation.

Infection and Alterations in Immunity and Inflammation

Reading Assignment: Infection and Alterations in Immunity and Inflammation
(Chapter 8)
Patients: Sally Begay, Room 304
Ira Bradley, Room 309

Before You Start

In this lesson, you will explore the effects of infection and immunodeficiency in two patients at Red Rock Canyon Medical Center. Read Chapter 8 in your textbook before you complete the following exercises. (You may find it helpful, however, to read through the questions in this lesson first, as a way to focus your reading.)

In the Supervisor's Office, sign in to work with Sally Begay for the Thursday 0700 shift. Go to the Nurses' Station and open her chart. Review the Physical & History, scrolling down to read all pages. Next, click on **Physicians' Orders** and review the orders for Sally Begay. Close her chart and access the EPR on the computer under the bookshelf. Open Sally Begay's EPR and review her laboratory results.

1. On admission, what viral infection was ruled out for Sally Begay?

2. From the information in her chart and laboratory results, what was her final diagnosis?

3. Read the discussion in your textbook about viral and bacterial infections. Compare and contrast bacterial infection and viral infection.

→ Return to Sally Begay's EPR. Click on **Vital Signs**, then on **Hematology**, and review the data in both these summaries.

   4. Which physical findings in Sally Begay's data support infection?

→ Your next task is to find out what medications have been prescribed for Sally Begay. You can get this information from two sources. One option is to reopen the patient's chart, click on **Physicians' Orders**, and review the medications that have been ordered for her. Another choice is to check the Medical Administration Record (MAR). To access the MAR, click on the blue notebook on the counter in the Nurses' Station. Then click on the tab with Sally Begay's room number—304—to review her medication record.

   5. What medications are being given to treat Sally Begay's infection?

Now review your textbook's discussions on deficiencies in immunity, especially the section on acquired immunodeficiency syndrome (AIDS).

6. What is the cause of AIDS?

7. Based on the material in your textbook, explain why there is no vaccine to prevent AIDS.

8. What populations are at risk for AIDS?

➡ Return to the Supervisor's Office and sign in to work with Ira Bradley for the Thursday 0700 shift. Go to the Nurses' Station, open his chart, and read the Physical & History. Now go to Ira Bradley's room. Click on **Health History**, then on **Health Perception**, and listen to the patient's responses in all three question categories.

9. Based on the data in his chart and the information gathered during the health history discussions with the nurse, does Ira Bradley have any documented risk behaviors for AIDS?

10. Using your textbook as a guide, describe the etiology and pathophysiology of AIDS.

11. Which of the clinical manifestations of AIDS does Ira Bradley exhibit?

→ Return to Ira Bradley's chart in the Nurses' Station. Review the physicians' orders and the expired MAR section.

12. What medications are being given to Ira Bradley to treat his HIV infection?

Stress and Disease

 Reading Assignment: Stress and Disease (Chapter 9)
Patients: Carmen Gonzales, Room 302
David Ruskin, Room 303
Sally Begay, Room 304
Ira Bradley, Room 309
Andrea Wang, Room 310

Before You Start

This lesson focuses on the connection between stress and disease. Before you begin these exercises, read Chapter 9 in your textbook. Keep your textbook nearby and work back and forth between text, CD, and this workbook to maximize your learning experience.

1. Chapter 9 in your textbook includes discussions of coping with stress and the general adaptation syndrome. After reviewing these discussions, list the three stages of the general adaptation syndrome.

Now apply what you have read about stress and the general adaptation syndrome to the five patients at Red Rock Canyon Medical Center. For each patient, sign in for the Thursday 1100 shift; then proceed to the Nurses' Station and review the patient's chart. Next, visit each patient and listen to his or her responses to the nurse's questions in the Coping/Stress category of the health history. Make notes as you listen.

2. Based on the data in the patient's charts and your observations of the Coping/Stress interviews, identify the stage of the general adaptation syndrome that best fits each patient.

→ Attend the Health Team meeting for Ira Bradley. Remember, you have to sign in to work with this patient before you can listen to the reports at the meeting. To find out where the meeting is being held, check the bulletin board in the Nurses' Station or move your cursor across the various rooms on the animated map in the upper right corner of your screen. After hearing the reports of all health team members, go to the Nurses' Station and open Ira Bradley's chart. Click on **Health Team** and read each member's written report.

3. What stressors can you identify for Ira Bradley and his family?

4. Discuss the effects of stress, coping, and Ira Bradley's illness trajectory.

📖 Review the information concerning stress-related disease in Table 9-4 of your textbook.

5. Which patients at Red Rock Canyon Medical Center have stress-related diseases or are at risk for stress-related disease? Explain.

6. Sally Begay is 58 years old. What effect will aging have on her immune system?

LESSON 9 ——————————————————

Biology of Cancer

——————————————————————————

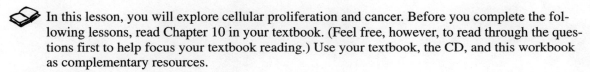 **Reading Assignment:** Biology of Cancer (Chapter 10)
Patient: Ira Bradley, Room 309

Before You Start

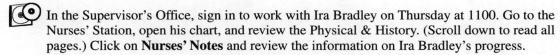 In this lesson, you will explore cellular proliferation and cancer. Before you complete the following lessons, read Chapter 10 in your textbook. (Feel free, however, to read through the questions first to help focus your textbook reading.) Use your textbook, the CD, and this workbook as complementary resources.

In the Supervisor's Office, sign in to work with Ira Bradley on Thursday at 1100. Go to the Nurses' Station, open his chart, and review the Physical & History. (Scroll down to read all pages.) Click on **Nurses' Notes** and review the information on Ira Bradley's progress.

1. Based on your review of Ira Bradley's chart, what kind of cancer does he have?

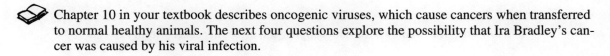 Chapter 10 in your textbook describes oncogenic viruses, which cause cancers when transferred to normal healthy animals. The next four questions explore the possibility that Ira Bradley's cancer was caused by his viral infection.

2. What viral infection does Ira Bradley have?

3. Based on the discussions in your textbook, explain the role of this virus (which you identified in question 2) in carcinogenesis.

4. Again referring to your textbook, identify and describe the two major groups of oncogenic viruses.

5. In which group of oncogenic viruses does HIV belong?

6. How does Ira Bradley's immunosuppression affect his susceptibility to cancer?

Tumor Invasion and Metastasis

 Reading Assignment: Tumor Invasion and Metastasis (Chapter 11)
Patients: Ira Bradley, Room 309

Before You Start

 In this lesson you will continue working with Ira Bradley, this time focusing on tumor invasion and metastasis. Before you begin the following exercises, read Chapter 11 in your textbook. As usual, keep your textbook nearby so that you can consult it when needed.

 To refamiliarize yourself with Ira Bradley's case, sign in to work with him on Friday at 1100 and review his chart in the Nurses' Station. Read the entire Physical & History. (Remember to scroll down to read all pages.)

1. Where is Ira Bradley's Kaposi's sarcoma located?

 2. Using your textbook as a guide, explain how Ira Bradley's Kaposi's sarcoma spreads locally.

3. Now focus on metastasis. Again referring to your textbook, explain how Ira Bradley's Kaposi's sarcoma metastasizes.

4. Think about what you have learned from Ira Bradley's Physical & History. Based on this data, does he have any signs and symptoms of local or metastatic spread?

5. What are the clinical manifestations of cancer? (Consult your textbook if necessary.)

→ Return to Ira Bradley's chart and again review his Physical & History, this time looking for clinical manifestations of cancer.

6. What clinical manifestations of cancer does Ira Bradley exhibit? (For help in answering this question, refer to the back inside cover of your textbook for normal laboratory values and contrast these with what you find in the laboratory data in the patient's chart.)

→ Once again, return to Ira Bradley's chart. This time, click on **Physicians' Orders** and **Expired MARs**, reviewing each section for medication orders.

7. Is Ira Bradley taking any of the chemotherapeutic drugs listed in Chapter 11 of your textbook? if so, which?

LESSON **11** ——————————————

Pain, Temperature Regulation, Sleep, and Sensory Function

———————————————————————

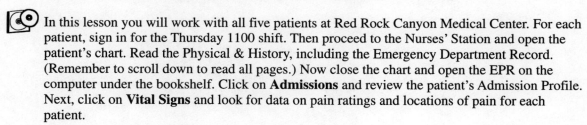

Reading Assignment: Pain, Temperature Regulation, Sleep, and Sensory Function (Chapter 14)

Patients: Carmen Gonzales, Room 302
David Ruskin, Room 303
Sally Begay, Room 304
Ira Bradley, Room 309
Andrea Wang, Room 310

Before You Start

Before you complete the exercises in this lesson, read Chapter 14 in your textbook (although you may want to review the questions first to focus your reading). Use your textbook, the CD, and this workbook as complementary resources to optimize your learning.

In this lesson you will work with all five patients at Red Rock Canyon Medical Center. For each patient, sign in for the Thursday 1100 shift. Then proceed to the Nurses' Station and open the patient's chart. Read the Physical & History, including the Emergency Department Record. (Remember to scroll down to read all pages.) Now close the chart and open the EPR on the computer under the bookshelf. Click on **Admissions** and review the patient's Admission Profile. Next, click on **Vital Signs** and look for data on pain ratings and locations of pain for each patient.

1. Which patients are experiencing pain? Where is their pain located?

2. Chapter 14 provides relevant discussions about pain. Using your textbook as a guide, summarize how pain is produced.

3. Refer to the discussions in Chapter 14 of your textbook on how aging may affect pain perception. Then apply this information to the case of Carmen Gonzales, who is 56 years old. Explain how her aging may affect her perception of pain.

4. Identify the physiologic responses to acute pain. (Consult your textbook if you need help.)

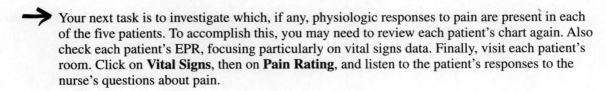 Your next task is to investigate which, if any, physiologic responses to pain are present in each of the five patients. To accomplish this, you may need to review each patient's chart again. Also check each patient's EPR, focusing particularly on vital signs data. Finally, visit each patient's room. Click on **Vital Signs**, then on **Pain Rating**, and listen to the patient's responses to the nurse's questions about pain.

5. Based on what you have learned by reading the chart and EPR data and by asking the patients about their pain, which—if any—physiologic responses to pain are present in each of the patients?

Return to the EPR and check each patient's vital signs data for evidence of fever. (Remember: For each patient, you will need to go back to the Supervisor's Office and sign in again by clicking the **Reset** icon before you can access that patient's EPR.)

6. Do any of the patients have fever? If so, describe the most probable reason for the fever.

7. Based on discussions in your textbook, what are the benefits of fever?

8. David Ruskin and Andrea Wang undergo surgery to repair their fractures. Describe the disorder of temperature regulation for which these patients are at risk during surgery.

→ Now visit each patient's room to observe the portion of the health history that addresses sleep and rest patterns. For each patient, sign in again for the Thursday 1100 shift. Inside the patient's room, click on **Health History**, then on **Sleep-Rest**, and listen to the nurse-patient discussions.

9. Which patients have trouble sleeping?

10. Based on your textbook reading, what effect does advancing age have on sleep patterns?

11. Aging also affects sensory function. What normal sensory changes would you expect to find in Carmen Gonzales based on her advancing age? (Describe specific physiological changes for each sensory organ affected.)

12. Does Carmen Gonzales exhibit any of these normal changes? (Review any data necessary to answer this question.)

LESSON 12

Concepts of Neurologic Dysfunction

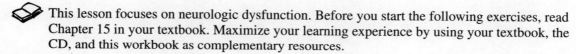 **Reading Assignment:** Concepts of Neurologic Dysfunction (Chapter 15)
Patients: David Ruskin, Room 303
Ira Bradley, Room 309
Andrea Wang, Room 310

Before You Start

This lesson focuses on neurologic dysfunction. Before you start the following exercises, read Chapter 15 in your textbook. Maximize your learning experience by using your textbook, the CD, and this workbook as complementary resources.

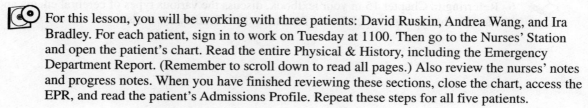 For this lesson, you will be working with three patients: David Ruskin, Andrea Wang, and Ira Bradley. For each patient, sign in to work on Tuesday at 1100. Then go to the Nurses' Station and open the patient's chart. Read the entire Physical & History, including the Emergency Department Report. (Remember to scroll down to read all pages.) Also review the nurses' notes and progress notes. When you have finished reviewing these sections, close the chart, access the EPR, and read the patient's Admissions Profile. Repeat these steps for all five patients.

1. Based on your review of patient data, do any of the patients have closed head injuries? If so, who?

2. Using your textbook as a guide, discuss the pathophysiology of acute confusional states.

3. From your reading of Chapter 15 in the textbook, what are the first clinical manifestations of acute confusional state?

4. Think again about two of the patients—Ira Bradley and David Ruskin. Which of the first clinical manifestations of acute confusion are documented for each of these patients?

5. For which alteration(s) in cerebral homeostasis are David Ruskin and Ira Bradley at risk?

6. Referring to Chapter 15 in your textbook, discuss the various types of cerebral edema and identify the type for which David Ruskin and Ira Bradley are at risk.

7. What clinical manifestations would you monitor in David Ruskin that would indicate developing cerebral edema?

8. Once again, consider the data you have reviewed for David Ruskin and Ira Bradley. Do these patients exhibit any of the clinical manifestations of cerebral edema? If so, which? (Return to these patient's charts and EPR summaries if necessary.)

9. Compare and contrast the problems of Andrea Wang, Ira Bradley, and David Ruskin. Do any of these patients have an alteration in motor function? If so, identify the patient(s) and explain what type of alteration is exhibited.

Alterations of Neurologic Function

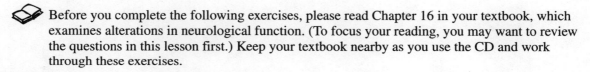

Reading Assignment: Alterations of Neurologic Function (Chapter 16)
Patients: David Ruskin, Room 303
    Ira Bradley, Room 309
    Andrea Wang, Room 310

Before You Start

Before you complete the following exercises, please read Chapter 16 in your textbook, which examines alterations in neurological function. (To focus your reading, you may want to review the questions in this lesson first.) Keep your textbook nearby as you use the CD and work through these exercises.

In this lesson, you will once again work with David Ruskin, Andrea Wang, and Ira Bradley. If necessary, refamiliarize yourself with these patients by signing in for the Thursday 1100 shift and reviewing the Physical & History in each patient's chart, including the Emergency Department Report. (Remember to scroll down to read all pages.)

1. Which patients have suffered head trauma?

2. Based on your reading of Chapter 16 in the textbook, describe the major causes of head trauma.

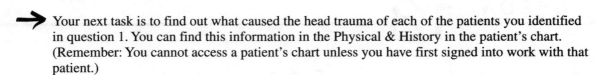 Your next task is to find out what caused the head trauma of each of the patients you identified in question 1. You can find this information in the Physical & History in the patient's chart. (Remember: You cannot access a patient's chart unless you have first signed into work with that patient.)

3. Describe the cause of each patient's head trauma.

 4. Based on your textbook reading, explain the pathophysiology of focal brain injury.

5. What symptoms of focal brain injury did David Ruskin exhibit in the emergency department?

6. Did Ira Bradley have any symptoms of focal brain injury in the emergency department? If so, what were they?

7. Which patient in Red Rock Canyon Medical Center has experienced spinal cord trauma?

8. Using your textbook as a guide, explain the pathophysiology of spinal cord injury.

9. Describe spinal shock.

10. What signs and symptoms of spinal shock did the patient you identified in question 7 exhibit in the emergency department? (If necessary, return to this patient's chart and review the Emergency Department Report in the Physical & History section.)

11. What occurrences mark the end of spinal shock?

→ Conduct a physical examination of the patient you identified in question 7. To do this, visit the patient's room, click on **Physical**, and then click on each of the three body areas. Observe the nurse's examination of all areas.

12. What data from the physical examination support resolving spinal shock in this patient?

13. For what life-threatening problem is this patient at risk after the spinal shock resolves?

14. Describe the pathophysiology of the problem you identified in question 13.

→ Continue working with the patient you identified in question 7. Leave the patient's room and return to the Nurses' Station. First access the EPR on the computer under the bookshelf and review the nursing assessment data for this patient by clicking on **Assessment**. Now close the EPR, open the patient's chart, and click on **Nurses' Notes**. Read the note for Thursday 0430.

15. Based on the EPR and chart data, what signs and symptoms of autonomic hyperreflexia (dysreflexia) does this patient exhibit?

16. What are the most common causes of autonomic hyperreflexia (dysreflexia)? (Consult your textbook for help.)

17. What was the cause of the patient's episode of autonomic hyperreflexia (dysreflexia)?

LESSON 14

Neurobiology of Schizophrenia, Mood Disorders, and Anxiety Disorders

 Reading Assignment: Neurobiology of Schizophrenia, Mood Disorders, and
Anxiety Disorders (Chapter 17)
Patients: Ira Bradley, Room 309
Andrea Wang, Room 310

Before You Start

Please read Chapter 17 in your textbook before you complete the following exercises. Work back and forth between the textbook, the CD, and this workbook to optimize your learning experience.

In this lesson you will work with two patients—Andrea Wang and Ira Bradley—focusing on issues related to depression and posttraumatic stress disorder. For each of the patients, sign in for 1100 on Thursday. Proceed to the Nurses' Station, open the patient's chart, and review the Physical & History, scrolling down to read all pages. Then close the chart, go to the patient's room, and listen to the entire health history interview. To do this, click on **Health History**; then click on each of the twelve health history categories and the three question areas for each category.

1. Based on the data you reviewed, which of these two patients has been diagnosed with depression?

2. Using your textbook as a guide, describe the etiology and pathophysiology of depression.

3. List the clinical manifestations of depression.

4. From your review of the patient's records and observations of the health history interview, what clinical manifestations of depression are exhibited by the patient you identified in question 1?

5. Based on your reading of Chapter 17 in the textbook, how is depression treated?

6. Describe the etiology and pathophysiology of posttraumatic stress disorder.

 7. What types of individuals are most vulnerable to posttraumatic stress disorder?

8. Based on her chart data and health history interview, does Andrea Wang fit the profile you described for question 7? Why or why not?

9. What are the symptoms of posttraumatic stress disorder?

10. Does Andrea Wang exhibit any of the symptoms of posttraumatic stress disorder? If so, which?

 11. Based on your reading of Chapter 17 in the textbook, how is posttraumatic stress disorder treated?

LESSON **15**

Alterations of Hormonal Regulation

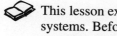 **Reading Assignment:** Alterations of Hormonal Regulation (Chapter 20)
Patient: Carmen Gonzales, Room 302

Before You Start

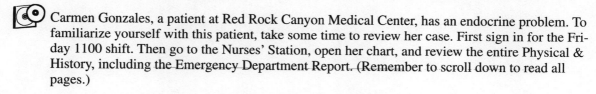 This lesson examines alterations in hormonal regulation and the consequences to physiologic systems. Before you complete this lesson, read Chapter 20 in your textbook. (Feel free, though, to review the questions in this lesson first. This will help focus your textbook reading.) To maximize your learning, use the textbook, the CD, and this workbook as complementary resources.

Carmen Gonzales, a patient at Red Rock Canyon Medical Center, has an endocrine problem. To familiarize yourself with this patient, take some time to review her case. First sign in for the Friday 1100 shift. Then go to the Nurses' Station, open her chart, and review the entire Physical & History, including the Emergency Department Report. (Remember to scroll down to read all pages.)

1. What alteration of hormonal regulation does Carmen Gonzales have?

 2. Based on your reading of Chapter 20 in the textbook, what endocrine organ is dysfunctioning in Carmen Gonzales' case?

3. Your textbook lists the criteria for diagnosis of diabetes mellitus. What are these criteria?

4. Describe the pathophysiology of type 2 diabetes mellitus.

→ Close Carmen Gonzales' chart and access her EPR on the computer under the bookshelf. Click on **Chemistry** and review the patient's blood glucose levels for the entire week.

5. Based on the EPR data, list Carmen Gonzales' blood glucose levels below by day and time.

Day	Time	Level

6. Are Carmen Gonzales' blood glucose levels within the normal range? (The normal serum glucose level is 70–110 mg/dl.) Do you notice any trends in her blood sugar levels?

→ In addition to blood glucose levels measured by laboratory tests, the nursing staff at Red Rock Canyon Medical Center assessed Carmen Gonzales' levels using the Accucheck system, a bedside blood glucose monitor. To find the values obtained from these measurements, click on **Vital Signs** in the EPR and check under "Blood Glucose."

7. List Carmen Gonzales' Accucheck blood glucose readings below by day and time.

Day	Time	Level

8. Now evaluate whether these bedside blood glucose readings are within the normal range. Are there any trends in these levels?

9. Based on the information in your textbook, what are the major risk factors for type 2 diabetes mellitus?

10. From your review of Carmen Gonzales' case, which of these risk factors does she have?

11. Review the characteristics of type 2 diabetes mellitus in Table 20-5 in your textbook. Which of these characteristics does Carmen Gonzales have?

12. List the four most frequently seen clinical manifestations of type 2 diabetes mellitus.

13. From what you have read about Carmen Gonzales' case, which of these manifestations does she have?

14. Using your textbook as a guide, list the nonspecific symptoms of type 2 diabetes mellitus.

15. Which of these nonspecific symptoms does Carmen Gonzales have?

→ Return to the Supervisor's Office and sign in to work with Carmen Gonzales on Thursday at 1100 so that you can observe her health history interviews. Go to her room, click **Health History**, and listen to her responses in each of the following categories: Activity, Nutrition-Metabolic, and Health Perception.

16. From what you heard during the health history discussions, what lifestyle changes would be beneficial to her condition?

17. Based on your knowledge of Carmen Gonzales' case, for what acute complications of diabetes mellitus is she at risk?

18. Using Chapter 20 in the textbook as your guide, what are the chronic complications of diabetes mellitus?

→ Go back to Carmen Gonzales' chart and again read her Physical & History, this time focusing on chronic complications of diabetes mellitus.

19. Based on the data in her chart, which of the chronic complications of diabetes mellitus does Carmen Gonzales have? What data documented in her chart support the presence of these complications?

LESSON — 16

Alterations of the Reproductive Systems

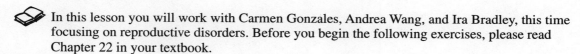

Reading Assignment: Alterations of the Reproductive Systems (Chapter 22)
Patients: Carmen Gonzales, Room 302
　　　　　Ira Bradley, Room 309
　　　　　Andrea Wang, Room 310

Before You Start

In this lesson you will work with Carmen Gonzales, Andrea Wang, and Ira Bradley, this time focusing on reproductive disorders. Before you begin the following exercises, please read Chapter 22 in your textbook.

In the Supervisor's Office, sign in to work with Carmen Gonzales on Thursday at 1100. Open her chart in the Nurses' Station and review the Physical & History, paying particular attention to data relevant to the reproductive system. (Remember to scroll down to read all the pages.) Also, observe the Health History Interviews, especially the nurse-patient discussions about Sexuality/Reproduction as well as the interview focused on Health Perception.

1. For what common reproductive infection is Carmen Gonzales at risk? Why?

2. Are there any data in the chart providing evidence that Carmen Gonzales has a vaginal infection or has had one in the past?

3. Based on your knowledge of Carmen Gonzales, is she at risk for undiagnosed cervical cancer? Why or why not?

4. Using your textbook as a guide, discuss the progressive nature of cervical cancer.

5. What are the symptoms of early cervical cancer?

6. How is cervical cancer diagnosed?

➡ Return to the Supervisor's Office. This time sign in to work with Andrea Wang for the Thursday 1100 shift. (Remember: You must click on **Reset** to select a new patient.) Find out where the health team meeting is being held for this patient by either checking the bulletin board in the Nurses' Station or moving your cursor across the animated map in the upper right corner of your screen. Go to that location, click on Andrea Wang's room number (310), and listen to each team member's report. Then open Andrea Wang's chart in the Nurses' Station, click on **Health Team**, and read the written reports. Close the chart and go to the patient's room. Click on **Health History** and observe the interviews focused on Sexuality/Reproduction and Role/Relationship.

7. What sexual concerns does Andrea Wang express?

8. Based on your reading of Chapter 22 in the textbook, what can you tell Andrea Wang about her prognosis for sexual function?

9. Using Chapter 22 in the textbook as your guide, list the causes of sexual dysfunction in men.

→ Once again, return to the Supervisor's Office to switch patients. Select Ira Bradley for the Thursday 0700 shift. Explore possible problems he may be having related to sexual dysfunction by doing the following:

- Attend Ira Bradley's health team meeting. Listen to each member's report.
- Read the Physical & History and the health team reports in the patient's chart.
- Visit Ira Bradley in his room and observe the health history interviews in the following categories: Sexuality/Reproductive and Role/Relationship.

10. What information do you find that suggests Ira Bradley's is experiencing sexual dysfunction?

LESSON 17

Sexually Transmitted Infections

 Reading Assignment: Sexually Transmitted Infections (Chapter 23)
Patient: Ira Bradley, Room 309

Before You Start

Before starting the following exercises, read Chapter 23, which focuses on sexually transmitted infections of the urogenital and other body systems. For this lesson, you will work with Ira Bradley, a patient with AIDS. As usual, organize your learning around combined use of your textbook, the CD, and this workbook.

1. Based on your reading of Chapter 23 in the textbook, is there a relationship between HIV and syphilis? Explain.

2. What are the symptoms of secondary syphilis?

Your next task is to apply what you have learned from your textbook to Ira Bradley's case. Sign in to work with him for the Tuesday 0700 shift. Open his chart in the Nurses' Station and review the Physical & History, scrolling down to read all pages. Also read the nurses' notes and physicians' notes, watching for symptoms of secondary syphilis. Close the chart and visit Ira Bradley in his room. Conduct a complete physical examination and obtain a full set of vital sign readings.

Now, take a virtual leap in time by returning to the Supervisor's Office and changing your shift to Thursday at 0700. (Keep Ira Bradley as your patient.) Review his chart, checking for updates since Tuesday. Once again, go to the patient's room and conduct a complete physical examination and vital signs measurement. Also observe health history interviews in the following areas: Sexuality/Reproduction, Role/Relationship, Health Perception, and Coping/Stress.

3. Based on your review of Ira Bradley's case, does he exhibit any of these symptoms? If so, which ones?

4. What laboratory tests would you like to evaluate to see whether Ira Bradley has syphilis?

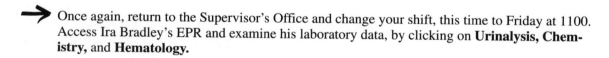 Once again, return to the Supervisor's Office and change your shift, this time to Friday at 1100. Access Ira Bradley's EPR and examine his laboratory data, by clicking on **Urinalysis, Chemistry,** and **Hematology.**

5. Can you find results for these tests?

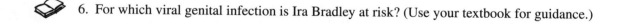 6. For which viral genital infection is Ira Bradley at risk? (Use your textbook for guidance.)

7. Describe the lesions that appear with the viral genital infection you identified in question 6.

8. Where would lesions of this viral infection be found?

9. Does Ira Bradley show evidence of this viral infection? (Review the patient's chart if necessary.)

10. For what systemic, sexually transmissible herpes virus is Ira Bradley at risk? (Use your textbook for guidance.)

11. How serious would such an infection be for this patient?

12. Is there any evidence in Ira Bradley's chart or from your physical examination data that he has the infection you identified in question 10?

Unit VIII—The Hematologic System

LESSON 18

Alterations of Erythrocyte Function

 Reading Assignment: Alterations of Erythrocyte Function (Chapter 25)
Patients: Carmen Gonzales, Room 302
David Ruskin, Room 303
Sally Begay, Room 304
Ira Bradley, Room 309
Andrea Wang, Room 310

Before You Start

This lesson examines anemia and other alterations in erythrocyte function. Read Chapter 25 in your textbook before you start the following exercises. Keep your textbook nearby so that you can consult it as you use the CD.

1. Using your textbook as a guide, what are the normal hematocrit and hemoglobin levels?

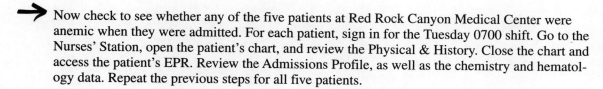 Now check to see whether any of the five patients at Red Rock Canyon Medical Center were anemic when they were admitted. For each patient, sign in for the Tuesday 0700 shift. Go to the Nurses' Station, open the patient's chart, and review the Physical & History. Close the chart and access the patient's EPR. Review the Admissions Profile, as well as the chemistry and hematology data. Repeat the previous steps for all five patients.

2. Based on your review of the data, which patient(s) had anemia on admission?

3. Review Table 25-3 and the normal blood count values on the back inside cover of your textbook. Compare these against the values of the patient(s) you listed in question 2. Which type of anemia does each patient have.

4. Based on your reading of Chapter 25 in the textbook, what are the clinical manifestations of each type of anemia you identified in question 3?

5. Once again, apply what you learned from your textbook to the patients in Red Rock Canyon Medical Center. Which of the clinical manifestations from question 4 are present in the patients who have anemia?

19

Alterations of Leukocyte, Lymphoid, and Hemostatic Function

Reading Assignment: Alterations of Leukocyte, Lymphoid, and Hemostatic Function (Chapter 26)

Patients: Carmen Gonzales, Room 302
David Ruskin, Room 303
Sally Begay, Room 304
Ira Bradley, Room 309
Andrea Wang, Room 310

Before You Start

This lesson examines alterations in leukocyte, lymphoid, and hemostatic function. Please read Chapter 26 in your textbook before you begin the following exercises. (Feel free, however, to review the questions first to focus your reading). Optimize your learning by using your textbook, the CD, and this workbook as complementary information resources.

Once again, you will be working with all five patients in Red Rock Canyon Medical Center. For each patient, sign in for the Tuesday 0700 shift; then go to one of the computers that allow you to access the EPRs. Open the patient's EPR and click on **Hematology**.

1. Evaluate the leukocyte levels of all five patients by completing these steps:

    a. In the table on the following page, record each patient's white blood cell count and differential counts from the earliest lab tests taken. Do this for all five patients.

    b. For each laboratory test listed, fill in the normal range of values in the second column of the table. Use the back inside cover of your textbook as a guide.

Lab Test	Normal Range of Values	Sally Begay	Ira Bradley	Carmen Gonzales	David Ruskin	Andrea Wang
WBC						
Neutrophil Segs						
Neutrophil Bands						
Monocytes						
Eosinophils						
Basophils						

2. Based on your review of the hematology data, which patients have leukocytosis?

3. From your reading of Chapter 26, which cells represent immature neutrophils?

4. Again based on your review of the hematology data, which patient exhibits a low neutrophil percentage? Explain what this finding means.

5. Which patient exhibits a high neutrophil percentage? What does this most likely indicate?

6. Identify the patient who exhibits a low lymphocyte percentage. What does this finding usually indicate?

7. Which patient exhibits a high lymphocyte percentage? Explain what this indicates.

8. One of the patients exhibits a high monocyte percentage. Who is this patient, and what does this finding most likely indicate?

9. Whose basophil percentage is high? Explain what this finding indicates.

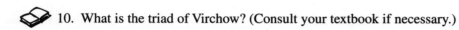 10. What is the triad of Virchow? (Consult your textbook if necessary.)

11. Which of the five patients is (are) at risk for thrombus formation? Explain why.

LESSON 20

Alterations of Cardiovascular Function

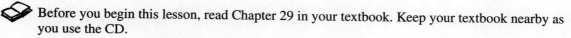 **Reading Assignment:** Alterations of Cardiovascular Function (Chapter 29)
Patients: Carmen Gonzales, Room 302
         Sally Begay, Room 304

Before You Start

Before you begin this lesson, read Chapter 29 in your textbook. Keep your textbook nearby as you use the CD.

Two patients at Red Rock Canyon Medical Center have a history of cardiovascular problems: Carmen Gonzales and Sally Begay. Your task is to gather data related to these patients' cardiovascular conditions using the resources available to you on the *Virtual Clinical Excursions* CD. As you conduct your search, take notes of any findings related to the pathophysiology of the cardiovascular system (use the space below). For each patient, sign in to work the Thursday 1100 shift. Next, access the EPR—either on the mobile computer in the hallway outside the Supervisor's Office or on the desktop computer under the bookshelf in the Nurses' Station. Search the EPR for any relevant data, especially blood pressure readings in the Admissions Profile and the vital signs summary.

Student Notes

Now go to the patient charts in the Nurses' Station. For both Sally Begay and Carmen Gonzales, review the chart data, especially the Physical & History section. (Remember to scroll down to read all pages.) Below, make note of any findings relevant to the cardiovascular system of these two patients.

Student Notes

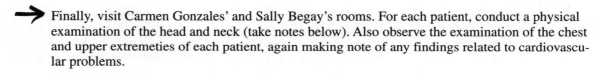 Finally, visit Carmen Gonzales' and Sally Begay's rooms. For each patient, conduct a physical examination of the head and neck (take notes below). Also observe the examination of the chest and upper extremeties of each patient, again making note of any findings related to cardiovascular problems.

Student Notes

1. Using Chapter 29 in your textbook as a guide, describe the pathophysiology of atherosclerosis.

2. What are the risk factors for atherosclerosis?

3. Now, based on what you have learned about Carmen Gonzales and Sally Begay, list and
describe any risk factors for atherosclerosis that you identified in either or both of these
patients.

4. What was each patient's blood pressure reading on admission?

5. Which of these patients has (have) hypertension based on the admission blood pressure reading?

6. Review your notes of each patients' serial blood pressure readings recorded in the vital signs summary in the EPR. Based on these findings, which of the patients has (have) hypertension? (If necessary, return to the EPR to check the exact readings again.)

7. For each patient you listed in your answer to question 6, identify the type of hypertension the patient has.

8. Using Chapter 29 in the textbook as your guide, what factors are associated with the type(s) of hypertension you identified in question 7.

9. Which of these factors does each patient listed in question 6 have?

10. What medication did each patient listed in question 6 take for hypertension prior to hospitalization?

11. Based on your reading of Chapter 29 in the textbook, what nonpharmacologic methods might be helpful in controlling the hypertension of the patient(s) you listed in question 6?

12. Once again, review your notes on Sally Begay and Carmen Gonzales. Which patient was previously diagnosed with coronary artery disease (CAD)?

13. List this patient's modifiable and nonmodifiable risk factors for CAD.

Modifiable   **Nonmodifiable**

14. Referring to Chapter 29 in your textbook, describe the association between menopause and CAD.

15. The patient you identified in question 12 is postmenopausal. What effect will that have on her CAD?

16. What could help slow the progression of this patient's CAD?

 17. Describe the three types of angina pectoris discussed in Chapter 29 of your textbook.

18. Based on these descriptions, what type of angina pectoris does Sally Begay have?

 19. You learned from Sally Begay's chart that she had a myocardial infarction 5 years ago. Using your textbook as a guide, describe the tissue changes that normally manifest in the infarcted area during each time period listed below.

Time Since Initial Incidence of MI	Tissue Changes
6–12 hours	
18–24 hours	
2–4 days	
4–10 days	
10–14 days	
6 weeks	

20. What complication(s) did Sally Begay develop after her myocardial infarction occurred?

21. Again, review the notes you took while reviewing Sally Begay's and Carmen Gonzales' data. Which of these patients has been diagnosed with congestive heart failure (CHF)? If necessary, return to each patient's chart to verify this information.

22. Using your textbook as a guide, list the signs and symptoms of congestive heart failure in the left column below. Now indicate which of these signs and symptoms you noted in Sally Begay and Carmen Gonzales by placing an **X** next to the sign/symptom under that patient's name.

Signs and Symptoms	Sally Begay	Carmen Gonzales

23. Reviewing your notes on Carmen Gonzales' data, list the signs and symptoms of right-sided heart failure seen in this patient. If necessary, return to the patient's chart and review the Physical & History and physicians' notes.

L E S S O N 21 ───────────────────────────────

Alterations of Pulmonary Function

───

 Reading Assignment: Alterations of Pulmonary Function (Chapter 32)
Patients: David Ruskin, Room 303
         Sally Begay, Room 304
         Ira Bradley, Room 309

Before You Start

For this lesson, review all the exercises first; then read Chapter 32 in your textbook. This should help focus your reading. To maximize your learning, keep your textbook nearby so that you can consult it during the lesson.

For questions 1 through 11 of this lesson, you will work with two patients—Ira Bradley and Sally Begay—both of whom have problems related to pulmonary function. For each patient, complete the following steps and use the space on the following page to take notes on any findings related to the pathophysiology of the pulmonary system:

- In the Supervisor's Office, sign in for the Tuesday 1100 shift.
- Review the EPR, paying special attention to these sections: Admissions Profile, assessment data, hematology data, and vital signs data (note, in particular, oxygen saturation and respiratory rate readings).
- Review the patient's chart, especially the Physical & History. (Remember to scroll down to read all pages.)
- Visit the patient's room and conduct a physical examination of the chest and upper extremities.

Student Notes on Ira Bradley

Student Notes on Sally Begay

1. Using the textbook as your guide, list the signs and symptoms of pulmonary disease below. Now, based on your review of Ira Bradley's and Sally Begay's data, indicate which signs and symptoms are present in each of these patients. Place an **X** under the patient's name next to each sign/symptom you noted.

Signs and Symptoms	Ira Bradley	Sally Begay

2. From the data you have reviewed, identify the chronic obstructive pulmonary disease (COPD) that is complicating Sally Begay's pneumonia.

3. Based on your analysis of the data in the patient chart and the COPD risk factors used in Chapter 32 of your textbook, what is the probable cause of Sally Begay's chronic obstructive pulmonary disease?

4. Referring again to Chapter 32 in your textbook, list the signs and symptoms that usually prompt patients with chronic bronchitis to seek medical care. Which of these are present in Sally Begay?

5. Using the textbook reading as your guide, define *pneumonia* and identify at-risk individuals. Which of these at-risk groups would include Sally Begay and/or Ira Bradley?

6. What are the microorganisms responsible for each of these patient's pneumonia?

7. Describe how pathogenic microorganisms can reach the lungs. (Consult your textbook if you need help.)

8. Based on your textbook reading, list the clinical manifestations of pneumonia below. Now review your notes on Ira Bradley and Sally Begay and identify which of these manifestation(s) each patient exhibits. Indicate this by placing an **X** under the patient's name next to each manifestation you noted. (Review the Physical & History and diagnostics sections of each patient's chart, as well as the EPR data.)

Clinical Manifestations	Ira Bradley	Sally Begay

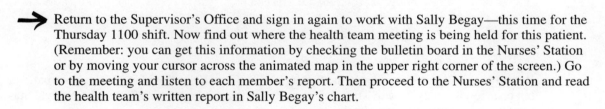 Return to the Supervisor's Office and sign in again to work with Sally Begay—this time for the Thursday 1100 shift. Now find out where the health team meeting is being held for this patient. (Remember: you can get this information by checking the bulletin board in the Nurses' Station or by moving your cursor across the animated map in the upper right corner of the screen.) Go to the meeting and listen to each member's report. Then proceed to the Nurses' Station and read the health team's written report in Sally Begay's chart.

9. What evidence can you cite from Sally Begay's data to support the health team's conclusion that she has inactive tuberculosis?

10. Is Ira Bradley at risk for tuberculosis? Why or why not? (If you are not sure, return to his chart and review the Physical & History section. Also consult your textbook for information on individuals with immunocompromised systems.)

11. Based on your reading of Chapter 32 in the textbook, what is the most common cause of acute pulmonary disease in hospitalized patients?

→ For the remaining questions in this lesson, sign in to work with a different patient, David Ruskin, for the Tuesday 0700 shift. Go to his chart in the Nurses' Station; click on **Diagnostics**, then on **Nurses' Notes,** reviewing each section.

12. Based on what you have read in David Ruskin's chart, what complication of impaired mobility and fracture could he develop?

13. Using your textbook as a guide, discuss the pathophysiology of pulmonary embolism.

Return to the sign-in computer in the Supervisor's Office. Keep David Ruskin as your patient, but change your duty time to Thursday at 1100. Once again, open his chart in the Nurses' Station, this time reviewing the physicians' notes and nurses' notes.

→ 14. Are there any symptoms documented in David Ruskin's chart that might lead you to suspect pulmonary embolism? If so, identify the symptom(s).

15. Based on your reading of Chapter 32 in the textbook, describe preventative measures that can be taken to prevent pulmonary embolism in the hospitalized patient.

LESSON **22** ——————————————

Alterations of Renal and Urinary Tract Function

———————————————————

 Reading Assignment: Alterations of Renal and Urinary Tract Function (Chapter 35)
Patients: Carmen Gonzales, Room 302
David Ruskin, Room 303
Sally Begay, Room 304
Ira Bradley, Room 309
Andrea Wang, Room 310

Before You Start

 Before you complete the following exercises, read Chapter 35 in your textbook. Be sure to use your textbook, the CD, and this workbook as complementary resources.

In the Supervisor's Office, sign in to work with Andrea Wang on Friday at 1100. Review her chart data in the Nurses' Station, keeping in mind the focus of this lesson—renal and urinary tract function.

1. Based on your textbook reading and what you have learned from Andrea Wang's chart, what obstructive disorder (related to renal and/or urinary tract function) is she at risk for following spinal cord injury?

2. Using Chapter 35 in your textbook as a guide, list below the types and causes of neurogenic bladder.

Type of Neurogenic Bladder	**Cause**

3. For which type of neurogenic bladder is Andrea Wang at risk?

4. Why is it important to diagnose and treat neurogenic bladder promptly?

5. Because of her neurogenic bladder, Andrea Wang is at risk for acute renal failure. List the types and causes of acute renal failure. (Use your textbook if you need help.)

Type	Causes

6. For which type of acute renal failure is Andrea Wang at risk?

7. Based on your textbook reading, what are the clinical manifestations of acute renal failure?

→ To complete the remaining exercises in this lesson, you will need to access the charts of the other four patients at Red Rock Canyon Medical Center. For each patient—Carmen Gonzales, David Ruskin, Sally Begay, and Ira Bradley—sign in for the Friday 1100 shift. Review the Physical & History section of each patient's chart and collect any information related to problems with renal function. Use the space below to take notes.

Student Notes

8. Based on your chart review, do any of these patients currently have urinary tract infections? If so, who?

9. Do any of the patients have a past history of urinary tract infections? If so, who?

10. Why are urinary tract infections rare in men?

11. Using Chapter 35 in the textbook as your guide, list and describe the clinical manifestations of cystitis.

12. Referring to the risk factors for cytosis identified in Chapter 35 of your textbook, which Red Rock Canyon Medical Center patients are at high risk for cystitis? Explain why.

13. Does Carmen Gonzales' type 2 diabetes mellitus put her at increased risk for chronic glomerulonephritis? Why or why not?

LESSON 23

Alterations of Digestive Function

Reading Assignment: Alterations of Digestive Function (Chapter 38)
Patients: Carmen Gonzales, Room 302
David Ruskin, Room 303
Sally Begay, Room 304
Ira Bradley, Room 309
Andrea Wang, Room 310

Before You Start

 Before you complete the following exercises, read Chapter 38 which examines how disorders of the gastrointestinal tract can disrupt one or more of its normal functions. Keep your textbook nearby and consult it often to reinforce your learning experience.

 You suspect that two patients—Carmen Gonzales and Ira Bradley—may have gastrointestinal dysfunction, but you need to investigate further to confirm this suspicion. To collect the necessary information, complete the following steps for each patient and use the space on the next page to take notes on any data related to gastrointestinal function:

- In the Supervisor's Office, sign in for the Tuesday 1100 shift.
- Review the Physical & History in the patient's chart. (Remember to scroll down to read all pages.)
- Access the EPR and review the patient's Admissions Profile.
- Visit the patient's room and listen to the nurse-patient discussions in the following categories of the health history: Nutrition-Metabolic, Activity, Elimination, and Health Perception.
- Conduct a physical examination of the patient's abdomen and lower extremities.

Student Notes

 1. Using Chapter 38 in the textbook as your guide, list the clinical manifestations of gastrointestinal dysfunction below. Now, based on what you have learned about Carmen Gonzales and Ira Bradley, indicate which of these manifestations each patient exhibits. Mark this by placing an **X** under the patient's name next to each manifestation you noted.

Clinical Manifestations	Carmen Gonzales	Ira Bradley

2. What disorder of nutrition does Carmen Gonzales have?

3. Referring to your textbook, list the disease processes associated with increased visceral fat. Based on your patient review, identify which of these disease processes Carmen Gonzales has.

4. How should Carmen Gonzales' nutritional disorder be treated?

5. What disorder of nutrition does Ira Bradley have?

 6. Based on your reading of Chapter 38 in the textbook, what are the pathologic causes of the disorder you identified in question 5? Which of these pathologic causes apply to Ira Bradley's nutritional disorder?

7. What treatment would be best for Ira Bradley's nutritional disorder?

 8. Another patient, David Ruskin, suffered a head injury following a bike accident. Referring to Chapter 38 in your textbook, name and define the type of ulcer seen in patients following severe head trauma.

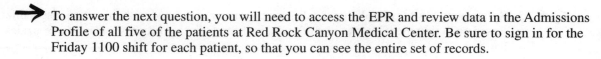

To answer the next question, you will need to access the EPR and review data in the Admissions Profile of all five of the patients at Red Rock Canyon Medical Center. Be sure to sign in for the Friday 1100 shift for each patient, so that you can see the entire set of records.

9. Using your text, create a list of risk factors for gallstones.

10. Based on your review of the Admissions Profile data, which of the five patients is at greatest risk for gallstones? Why?

LESSON **24**

Alterations of Musculoskeletal Function

Reading Assignment: Alterations of Musculoskeletal Function (Chapter 41)
Patients: Carmen Gonzales, Room 302
David Ruskin, Room 303
Andrea Wang, Room 310

Before You Start

Chapter 41 in the textbook presents a review of musculoskeletal injuries, as well as discussions of alterations in bones, joints, and muscles that result from various disorders. To focus your reading, review the questions in this lesson before you read the chapter. Be sure to use the information resources available in your textbook and the CD as you work through these exercises.

1. Below and on the next page, list typical complete and incomplete fractures. For each fracture, provide a definition or description. Use your texbook for help.

Complete Fractures	Definition or Description

Incomplete Fractures	Definition or Description

 Two patients, David Ruskin and Andrea Wang, have fractures. Your task is to learn as much as you can about these fractures. First sign in to work with David Ruskin on Thursday at 0700. Access his chart in the Nurses' Station and review the Physical & History, scrolling down to read all pages. Now click on **Diagnostics** and review that section for data related to alterations in musculoskeletal function. (Keep notes below.) Finally, visit David Ruskin's room and conduct a complete physical examination, again keeping notes.

Now repeat the previous steps for Andrea Wang.

Student Notes

2. Based on the data you have gathered, what type of fracture does David Ruskin have?

3. What type of fracture does Andrea Wang have?

4. Below, list the clinical manifestations of fracture. (Refer to your textbook if necessary.) Then identify those manifestations found in Andrea Wang and David Ruskin. Indicate this by placing an **X** under the patient's name next to each manifestation you noted.

Clinical Manifestations	**Andrea Wang**	**David Ruskin**

 5. Based on your reading of Chapter 41, list the three methods for fracture reduction.

6. Which of these methods was (were) used on David Ruskin?

7. Which of these methods was (were) used on Andrea Wang?

8. In addition to the fracture, what other tissues were injured in David Ruskin's arm?

9. David Ruskin has suffered severe muscle trauma. What life-threatening complication might he develop?

10. How would you monitor for this problem?

11. Referring to your textbook, list the causes of secondary muscular dysfunction.

12. Based on the notes you collected from Andrea Wang's data, identify and describe the causes of the secondary muscle dysfunction she is experiencing.

Return to the Supervisor's Office and sign in to work with Carmen Gonzales on Thursday at 1100. Gather as much data as you can related to this patient's musculoskeletal dysfunction by completing the following steps and keeping notes below:

- Access her EPR and review her Admissions Profile.
- Conduct a physical examination of Carmen Gonzales' abdomen and lower extremities.
- Review her chart, especially the diagnostic reports and the Physical & History section.

Student Notes

13. Based on your review, what infectious bone disease does Carmen Gonzales have?

14. Why is this bone disease difficult to treat? (Consult your textbook if you need help.)

15. What microorganisms cause the infectious bone disease that Carmen Gonzales has?

16. Referring to discussions in Chapter 41, name and define the two types of osteomyelitis. Which type does Carmen Gonzales have?

17. Using your textbook as a guide, list the clinical manifestations of osteomyelitis. Identify those present in Carmen Gonzales by placing an **X** next to each manifestation you noted in her records.

Clinical Manifestations   **Carmen Gonzales**

18. List the treatment options for osteomyelitis and place an **X** next to those used for Carmen Gonzales.

Treatments   **Carmen Gonzales**

LESSON 25

Structure, Function, and Disorders of the Integument

 Reading Assignment: Structure, Function, and Disorders of the Integument
(Chapter 43)

Patients: Carmen Gonzales, Room 302
David Ruskin, Room 303
Sally Begay, Room 304
Ira Bradley, Room 309
Andrea Wang, Room 310

Before You Start

The skin covers the entire body and is considered the largest organ of the body. Chapter 43 in your textbook focuses on the structure and function of the integumentary system, as well as disorders of this system. Read this chapter before you complete the following exercises. Remember to use your textbook, the CD, and this workbook as complementary information resources.

1. Based on your textbook reading, name and describe the two layers of skin.

In the Supervisor's Office, sign in to work with David Ruskin on Tuesday at 0700. Open his chart in the Nurses' Station and review the Physical & History, focusing particularly on the Emergency Department Report. (Remember to scroll down to read all pages.) Determine the location and extent of abrasions David Ruskin suffered in his accident.

2. Abrasions are classed as what type of secondary skin lesion?

→ Return to the Supervisor's Office and sign in to work the Tuesday 0700 shift, this time selecting Andrea Wang as your patient. Go to the Nurses' Station and review her entire chart, paying attention for any data relevant to the integumentary system. Then access her EPR and note any findings related to skin condition in the assessment data summary.

3. Describe the pressure-induced skin dysfunction for which Andrea Wang is at risk following her spinal cord injury. Based on your review of her chart and EPR data, is there any evidence that Andrea Wang had this skin dysfunction on Tuesday morning?

→ Now sign in to work with Carmen Gonzales at 0700 on Tuesday. First, review her chart data. Then go to her room to conduct a physical examination of her lower extremities. Remember, to do this, enter her room, click on **Physical,** and then click on **Abdomen and Lower Extremities.**

4. What skin infection does Carmen Gonzales have surrounding her wound?

→ Expand your knowledge base of Carmen Gonzales' leg wound by consulting the assessment data summary in her EPR.

5. What are the signs and symptoms of the infection you identified in question 4? Which of these does Carmen Gonzales exhibit?

→ To complete questions 6 through 15, you will need to review the data available on the remaining patients—Ira Bradley and Sally Begay. First read through these questions to focus your review. For each patient, sign in for the Tuesday 0700 shift. Review the Physical & History in the patient's chart, as well as the assessment data in the EPR.

6. Using your textbook as a guide, list the risk factors for candidiasis.

7. Which of the five patients has candidiasis? What type of candidiasis does this patient have? Explain why this patient is particularly susceptible to this infection.

8. Based on your understanding of candidiasis, which of the other patients are at risk for this infection, and why? (Return to the patients' charts if necessary.)

9. Referring to Chapter 43 in your textbook, list the risk factors for skin cancer.

10. Based on the data you have reviewed, which of the patients is (are) at greatest risk for skin cancer? Explain.

11. What areas of the skin are at greatest risk for skin cancer?

12. Name and describe the most common type of skin cancer.

13. One of the patients, Sally Begay, works outdoors. How can she help to minimize her chances of getting basal cell carcinoma?

 14. What type of skin cancer does Ira Bradley have? Describe this condition, including presentations, causes, characteristics, and clinical manifestations. Also identify, describe, and differentiate the two forms of this skin cancer. (Refer to your textbook if necessary.) Which form does Ira Bradley most likely have? Explain.

15. Using Chapter 43 in your textbook, define and describe keloids. Identify which patients at Red Rock Canyon Medical Center are at risk to develop them and explain why.

LESSON **26** ————————————————

Shock, Multiple Organ Dysfunction Syndrome, and Burns in Adults

 Reading Assignment: Shock, Multiple Organ Dysfunction Syndrome, and Burns in Adults (Chapter 45)

Patients: Carmen Gonzales, Room 302
David Ruskin, Room 303
Sally Begay, Room 304
Ira Bradley, Room 309
Andrea Wang, Room 310

Before You Start

Chapter 45 explores the pathophysiology of shock and multiple organ dysfunction, as well as the complications resulting from burns and smoke inhalation. Read this chapter before you begin the following exercises, although you may want to review the questions first to help guide your reading. Work back and forth between textbook, CD, and workbook, using them as complementary information resources.

For this lesson, you will work with all five patients at Red Rock Canyon Medical Center. Your first responsibility is to familiarize yourself with their cases in order to set priorities for care, as well as monitor for complications. You are presently concerned with patient problems related to potential shock and possible multiple organ dysfunction. With that in mind, sign in for each patient, selecting the Friday 1100 shift. Review the patient's chart—particularly the Physical & History, nurses' notes, and physicians' notes. (Remember to scroll down to read all pages.) As you conduct your review, use the space on the next page to take notes on findings related to the potential for shock and multiple organ dysfunction syndrome.

Student Notes

1. Using Chapter 45 in the textbook as your guide, describe cardiogenic shock.

2. Which of the patients is (are) at risk for cardiogenic shock? Explain why.

3. What clinical manifestations of cardiogenic shock should you watch for in the patient(s) you identified in question 2?

4. Name and describe the type of shock present in Andrea Wang on her arrival at the Emergency Department.

5. List the clinical manifestations of the type of shock you identified in question 4. Are any of these manifestations documented as present in Andrea Wang in the Emergency Department Record? If so, which?

6. What is the treatment for this type of shock? When did Andrea Wang receive this treatment?

7. Based on your reading of Chapter 45 in the textbook, describe how an infection can cause a patient to deteriorate into septic shock.

8. Identify the patient(s) at risk for septic shock.

9. Using Chapter 45 as your guide, list all the risk factors for multiple organ dysfunction syndrome (MODS).

10. Which of the five patients is (are) at risk for MODS? Why?

Answers

Lesson 1—Cellular Biology

1. **Movement:** Muscle cells can generate forces that produce motion. Muscles that are attached to bones produce limb movements, whereas those that enclose hollow tubes or cavities move or empty contents when they contract. For example, the contraction of smooth muscle cells surrounding blood vessels changes the diameter of the vessels; the contraction of muscles in walls of the urinary bladder expels urine.

   Conductivity: Conduction as a response to a stimulus is manifested by a wave of excitation, an electrical potential, that passes along the surface of the cell to reach its other parts. Conductivity is the chief function of nerve cells.

   Metabolic absorption: All cells take in and use nutrients and other substances from their surroundings. Cells of the intestine and the kidney are specialized to carry out absorption. Cells of the kidney tubules reabsorb fluids and synthesize proteins. Intestinal epithelial cells reabsorb fluids and synthesize protein enzymes.

   Secretion: Certain cells, such as mucous gland cells, can synthesize new substances from substances they absorb and can secrete the new substances to serve as needed elsewhere. Cells of the adrenal gland, testis, and ovary can secrete hormonal steroids.

   Excretion: All cells can rid themselves of waste products resulting from the metabolic breakdown of nutrients. Membrane-bound sacs (lysosomes) within cells contain enzymes that break down, or digest, large molecules, turning them into waste products that are released from the cell.

   Respiration: Cells absorb oxygen, which is used to transform nutrients into energy in the form of adenosine triphosphate (ATP). Cellular respiration, or oxidation, occurs in organelles called *mitochondria*.

   Reproduction: Tissue growth occurs as cells enlarge and reproduce themselves. Even without growth, tissue maintenance requires that new cells be produced to replace cells that are lost normally through cellular death. Not all cells are capable of continuous division, and some cells, such as nerve cells, cannot reproduce.

   Communication: Communication is critical for all the other functions above that enable the survival of the society of cells. Pancreatic cells, for instance, secrete and release insulin to tell muscle cells to take up sugar from the blood for energy. Constant communication allows the maintenance of a dynamic steady state.

2. Andrea Wang could have alterations in all cellular functions following her spinal cord injury. David Ruskin could have alterations in movement and conductivity following his fracture. Ira Bradley could have alterations in all cellular functions because of his end-stage HIV infection. Sally Begay could have alterations in movement because of her CAD, alterations in respiration because of her COPD and TB, and alterations in metabolic absorption

and reproduction because of her infection. Carmen Gonzales could have alterations in all cellular functions because of her type 2 diabetes mellitus. Additionally, she could have alterations in movement because of her CAD, alterations in respiration because of her CHF, and alterations in metabolic absorption and reproduction because of her infection.

3. Carmen Gonzales, Ira Bradley, and Sally Begay

4. Cellular receptors are protein molecules on the plasma membrane, in the cytoplasm, or in the nucleus that are capable of binding with specific smaller molecules. Receptors for infectious organisms—or antigen receptors—bind bacteria, viruses, and parasites. Antigen receptors on white blood cells recognize and bind with antigenic microorganisms and activate the immune and inflammatory responses.

5. All of them

6. **Phase 1:** Large molecules are broken down into their smaller substrates—proteins into amino acids, polysaccharides into simple sugars, fats into fatty acids and glycerol. These processes are called *digestion* and occur outside the cell by the action of secreted enzymes.
   Phase 2: Smaller molecules enter the cells and are further broken down in the cytoplasm. The most important action is the lysis of glucose—glucolysis—which produces 2 ATP molecules per glucose molecule. Pyruvate is also broken down in the mitochondria to the acetyl group of acetyl-CoA, which release energy when hydrolyzed.
   Phase 3: The acetyl group of acetyl-CoA is completely degraded to CO and H_2O. Most ATP is generated in this phase, which begins with the Kreb's cycle and ends with oxidative phosphorylation.

7. Cellular intake and output occurs by different mechanisms, depending on the characteristics of the substance to be transported. Water and small, electrically uncharged molecules move easily through pores in the plasma membrane's lipid bilayer. This process is called *passive transport* and will occur naturally through any semipermeable barrier and does not require any expenditure of energy by the cell. Passive transport is driven by osmosis, hydrostatic pressure, and diffusion, all of which depend on the laws of physics and do not require life. Larger molecules move into the cell by the mechanism of mediated transport, which can be active or passive and requires the expenditure of cellular energy. Endocytosis and excocytosis are forms of active transport using vesicle formation.

8. David Ruskin and Andrea Wang

9. Carmen Gonzales, Ira Bradley, and Andrea Wang

10. Reproduction requires two sequential phases—mitosis (nuclear division) and cytokinesis (cytoplasmic division). There are four phases of the cell cycle:
    - S (synthesis) phase, in which DNA is synthesized in the cell nucleus.
    - G_2 (gap) phase, in which RNA and protein synthesis occurs.
    - M (mitosis) phase, which includes both nuclear and cytoplasmic division.
    - G_1 (gap) phase, which is the period between the M phase and the start of DNA synthesis. Interphase (composed of the G phases and the M phase) is the longest phase of the cell cycle. The M phase of the cell cycle begins with prophase, during which each chromosome produces two identical halves (chromatids) attached to each other by a centromere. The nuclear membrane surrounding the nucleus disappears. Spindle fibers on both sides of the cell pull the chromosomes to opposite sides. During metaphase (the next phase), the spindle fibers begin to pull the centromeres of the chromosomes. Anaphase begins when the centromeres are pulled apart and the chromatids are separated. By the end of this phase, 46 chromosomes are lying on each side of the cell. During the next phase, telophase, spindle fibers disappear and new nuclear membranes form around each group of 46 chromosomes. The cytoplasm divides roughly in half, and two diploid or daughter cells form from the original cell. Rates of cellular division vary among different types of cells and can take hours,

days, or years. The time spent in the G_1 phase determines the length of time for the cell cycle.

11. Ira Bradley has the greatest nutritional need since he is at the end stage of his disease and because the candidiasis in his mouth has made it difficult for him to swallow. This has resulted in a decreased intake; thus he is underweight, dehydrated, and malnourished.

Lesson 2—Altered Cellular and Tissue Biology

1. Andrea Wang's lower extremities will soon show signs of atrophy because of her spinal cord injury.

2. Atrophy is a decrease or shrinkage of cellular size. It can affect any organ, but most commonly affects skeletal muscle, the heart, secondary sex organs, and the brain. The causes of atrophy include a decrease in workload, use, blood supply, nutrition, hormonal stimulation, and nervous stimulation. Individuals immobilized in bed for a prolonged time exhibit a type of skeletal muscle atrophy called *disuse syndrome*. The atrophic muscle cell contains less endoplasmic recticulum and fewer mitochondria and myofilaments than does the normal cell. In muscular atrophy caused by nerve loss, oxygen consumption and amino acid uptake are rapidly reduced. The biochemical changes of atrophy are not well understood, but mechanisms probably include decreased protein synthesis, increased protein catabolism, or both.

3. Carmen Gonzales and Sally Begay

4. Hypertrophy is an increase in the size of the cells and, consequently, in the size of the affected organ. The cells of the heart and kidneys are particularly responsive to enlargement. The increase in cellular size is associated with an increased accumulation of protein in the cellular components, not with an increase in cellular fluid. The exact physiologic mechanism of hypertrophy in various cells remains uncertain. Muscular hypertrophy might involve an increase in the rate of protein synthesis, a decrease in the rate of protein degradation, or both. If protein degradation decreases and the rate of protein synthesis is normal or slightly increased, the net effect is an accumulation of cellular protein. In myocardial hypertrophy, initial enlargement is caused by dilation of the cardiac chambers, but this is short lived and is followed by increased synthesis of cardiac muscle proteins, allowing muscle fibers to do more work. The nucleus is also hypertrophic with increased synthesis of DNA. Although fully matured muscle cells are unable to undergo further mitosis, they are capable of increased DNA synthesis. Why cardiac muscle cells are unable to progress through the cell cycle to mitosis is unclear. Eventually, however advanced hypertrophy can lead to myocardial failure. Muscular hypertrophy tends to diminish if the excessive workload diminishes.

5. Hypoxic cellular injury

6. Hypoxia, a lack of sufficient oxygen, is the single most common cause of cellular injury. The most common cause of hypoxia is ischemia, reduced blood flow. A gradual narrowing of arteries (arteriosclerosis) and complete blockage often cause ischemic injury by blood clots (thrombosis). Progressive hypoxia caused by gradual arterial obstruction is better tolerated than a sudden acute obstruction resulting in anoxia, a total lack of oxygen. An acute obstruction in a coronary artery can cause myocardial cell death within minutes if the blood supply is not restored, whereas gradual onset of ischemia usually results in myocardial adaptation. Within 1 minute of anoxia, myocardial cells become pale and have difficulty contracting; within 3 to 5 minutes, contraction stops. Restoration of blood supply, or reperfusion, can cause additional injury because of free radicals. Cellular death is caused by an accumulation of calcium in the mitochondria.

7. Sally Begay suffered a myocardial infarction 5 years ago. She also has a history of stable angina.

8. Ira Bradley

9. Essential nutrients—proteins, carbohydrates, lipids, vitamins, and minerals—are required for cells to function normally. Protein deficiency causes a decrease in the intestinal mucosal mass (resulting in decreased absorptive function), affects the integrity of the pancreas (resulting in diminished exocrine secretion), and causes interstitial edema. Carbohydrate deficiency causes metabolism of fats, as does lipid deficiency. Vitamin and mineral deficiencies impair cellular functioning and can cause abnormalities in chromosomes and in DNA synthesis.

10. Because of Ira Bradley's end-stage disease process and his limited oral intake, he is at risk for deficiencies in all essential nutrients.

11. Three patients have increased melanin because of their ethnicity—David Ruskin, who is African-American, Carmen Gonzales, who is Hispanic, and Sally Begay, who is Native American.

12. Melanin, a brown-black pigment derived from the amino acid tyrosine, accumulates in the epithelial cells of the skin and retina. It is extremely important because it protects the skin against long exposure to sunlight and is considered an essential factor in the prevention of skin cancer. Ultraviolet light stimulates the synthesis of melanin, which probably absorbs ultraviolet rays during subsequent exposure. Melanin also may protect the skin by trapping the injurious free radicals produced by the action of ultraviolet light and skin.

13. Carmen Gonzales has necrosis and gangrene on her lower left leg.

14. Cellular death leads to the process of cellular dissolution, called *necrosis*. Necrosis is the sum of cellular changes after local cell death and the process of cellular self-digestion, known as *autodigestion*, or *autolysis*. The structural signs that indicate irreversible injury and progression to necrosis are the dense clumping and progressive disruption of genetic material and the disruption of the plasma and organelle membranes. In the later stages of necrosis, most organelles are disrupted, and karolysis (nuclear dissolution from the action of hydrolytic enzymes) is underway. In some cells the nucleus shrinks and becomes a small, dense mass of genetic material—a process called *pyknosis*. The pyknotic nucleus eventually dissolves as a result of the action of hydrolytic lysosomal enzymes on DNA. Different types of necrosis tend to occur in different organs or tissues and sometimes can indicate the mechanism or cause of cellular injury. The four major types of necrosis are coagulative, liquefactive, caseous, and fatty.

    Another type, gangrenous necrosis, is not a distinctive type of cell death but a reference to larger areas of tissue death. *Gangrenous necrosis*, a term commonly used in surgical clinical practice, refers to death of tissue and results from severe hypoxic injury, commonly occurring because of atherosclerosis (or blockage) of major arteries, especially in the lower leg. With hypoxia and subsequent bacterial invasion, the tissues can undergo necrosis. Dry gangrene is usually a result of coagulative necrosis. The skin dries significantly and shrinks (resulting in wrinkles), and skin color changes to dark brown or black. Wet gangrene develops when neutrophils invade the site, causing liquefactive necrosis. This usually occurs in internal organs, causing the site to become cold, swollen, and black. A foul odor is present, produced by pus, and if systemic symptoms become severe, death can ensue. Gas gangrene, a special type of gangrene, is caused by infection of injured tissue by one of the many species of *Clostridium*. These anaerobic bacteria produce hydrolytic enzymes and toxins that destroy connective tissue and cellular membranes and cause bubbles of gas to form in muscle cells. Gas gangrene can be fatal if enzymes lyse the membranes of red blood cells, destroying their oxygen-carrying capacity. Death is a result of shock. The condition is treated with antitoxins and supplemental oxygen delivered in a hyperbaric (pressurized) chamber.

15. Dry gangrene with underlying infection, causing pus

Lesson 3—The Cellular Environment: Fluids and Electrolytes, Acids and Bases

1. The presence of edema

2. Edema is the accumulation of fluid within the interstitial spaces. It is a problem of fluid distribution and does not necessarily indicate fluid excess. The pathophysiologic process is related to an increase in the forces favoring fluid filtration from the capillaries or lymphatic channels into the tissues. The most common mechanisms include increased hydrostatic pressure, decreased plasma oncotic pressure, increased capillary membrane permeability, and lymphatic obstruction. In David Ruskin's case, the mechanism is the increased capillary permeability due to inflammation (a normal response to trauma) at the fracture site. Disrupted vasculature may also contribute to leakage of fluid into the interstitial spaces.

3. On Sunday at 0800, Sally Begay's serum potassium level was 3.3 mEq/l. Normal level is 3.5 to 5.5 mEq/l. Her potassium level is below normal, indicating hypokalemia.

4. Hydrochlorothiazide, a thiazide diuretic, inhibits the reabsorption of sodium chloride, thus causing a diuretic effect. The distal tubular flow rate in the kidneys promotes increased potassium excretion. If sodium loss is severe, the compensating aldosterone secretion may further deplete potassium stores.

5. Sally Begay should eat foods rich in potassium and take a potassium supplement.

6. Yes. Ira Bradley's serum potassium level was elevated—5.7 mEq/l. This condition is called *hyperkalemia*.

7. The most common characteristics of hyperkalemia are muscle weakness and changes in the electrocardiogram. Mild attacks cause increased neuromuscular irritability, which may be manifested as tingling in the lips and fingers, restlessness, intestinal cramping, and diarrhea. Hyperkalemia could be contributing to Ira Bradley's extreme weakness and diarrhea.

8. 135 to 147 mEq/l

9. It is 152 mEq/l = increased = hypernatremia.

10. Hypernatremia may be caused by an acute gain in sodium or a loss of water. Increased sodium in relation to water loss is associated with fever or respiratory infections, which increase respiratory rate and enhance water loss from the lungs. Ira Bradley's vital signs data and his Physical & History reveal an elevated temperature and a pulmonary infection, which would both contribute to his hypernatremia. Additionally, he has had difficulty with fluid intake because of pain with swallowing.

11. With increasing age the percentage of total body water declines. This decrease is caused in part by an increased amount of fat and a decreased amount of muscle and by the reduced ability to regulate sodium and water balance. With age the kidneys become less efficient in producing concentrated urine, and the responses for conserving sodium become sluggish. The normal reduction of total body water in older adults becomes clinically important in the presence of stress, such as fever of dehydration from any cause. Loss of body fluids at such times can be severe and life-threatening.

12. Respiratory acidosis

13. Respiratory acidosis occurs when ventilation is depressed. Carbon dioxide is retained, increasing hydrogen ions and producing acidosis. Common causes include depression of the respiratory center, respiratory muscle paralysis, disorders of the chest wall, and disorders of the lung parenchyma. If Andrea Wang develops spinal shock, she may exhibit some respiratory muscle paralysis, leading to the development of respiratory acidosis.

Lesson 4—Genes, Environment, and Common Diseases

1.

Patient	Disorder	General Risk Factors	Patient's Risk Factors
Sally Begay	Coronary artery disease	Obesity, cigarette smoking, hypertension, elevated cholesterol level, and positive family history (usually defined as having one affected first-degree relative)	Has slightly elevated blood pressure and has a positive history (her mother)
Carmen Gonzales	Coronary artery disease	Obesity, cigarette smoking, hypertension, elevated cholesterol level, and positive family history (usually defined as having one affected first-degree relative)	Is mildly obese, has slightly elevated diastolic blood pressure, and may have a positive family history
Carmen Gonzales	Type 2 diabetes mellitus	Obesity and positive family history	Is mildly obese and believes her mother had diabetes

2. Carmen Gonzales

3. Obesity is a risk factor for heart disease, stroke, and type 2 diabetes mellitus.

4.

Patient	At Risk For	Has Already Developed
Sally Begay	Type 2 diabetes mellitus	Coronary artery disease; hypertension
Carmen Gonzales		Type 2 diabetes mellitus; coronary artery disease
Ira Bradley	None	None
Andrea Wang	Hypertension; type 2 diabetes mellitus	None
David Ruskin	Coronary artery disease; type 2 diabetes mellitus	None

Lesson 5—Immunity

1. The normal immune system is continually challenged by a spectrum of chemical substances that it recognizes as foreign; these are called *antigens*. Some antigens are infectious agents, and some are noninfectious substances from the environment. The body's reaction to antigenic challenges is the immune response, in which physiologic and biochemical interactions cause the maturation and activation of two types of immunocytes—B lymphocytes and T lymphocytes. These lymphocytes act in different ways to recognize and destroy specific antigens. Individual B and T cells recognize only one specific antigen. The B cells produce antibodies, which incapacitate the antigen. The T cells attach to the antigen directly. Once B and T cells have been exposed to a particular antigen, some of them, called *memory cells*, become capable of remembering the antigen and of acting even faster if that antigen invades

the host again. The immune response can be amplified or suppressed by both exogenous and endogenous modulators.

2. Carmen Gonzales

3. She has had two major infections in the past 5 months.

4. Immune function decreases in advanced age. T cell function and specific antibody responses to antigenic challenge diminish; yet there is an increase in levels of circulating autoantibodies (antibodies against self-antigens) and immune complexes. In addition, there is an increased incidence of spontaneous monoclonal antibody production without concurrent B cell malignancy (myeloma). By 45 to 50 years of age, thymic size is only 15% of maximum. The level of thymic hormone production and the capacity of the thymus to mediate T cell differentiation decreases with thymic atrophy. Numbers of T cells do not decrease with age, but T cell function may deteriorate. Individuals over 60 years of age generally exhibit decreased delayed hypersensitivity response, decreased T cell–mediated responses to infections, and decreased T cell activity.

5. Ira Bradley

6. Lymphocyte

7. B lymphocyte

8. T lymphocyte

9. Ira Bradley

10. The major effects of the cell-mediated immune response are:
    - Cytotoxicity—Cytotoxic T cells mediate the direct, cellular killing of target cells, such as virally infected cells, tumors, and foreign grafts. This function requires cellular contact, binding, and release of toxic substances from the Tc cell.
    - Delayed hypersensitivity—Td cells are involved in the inflammatory response and produce soluble mediators (lymphokines) that influence other cells, such as macrophages.
    - Memory—Memory cells are responsible for the accelerated response to a second antigenic challenge (the secondary immune response).
    - Control—Helper T cells facilitate and suppressor T cells inhibit both humoral and cell-mediated immune responses.

11. The diagnosis of HIV/AIDS, fever, recurring severe opportunistic infections (*Pneumocystis carinii* pneumonia, candidiasis), Kaposi's sarcoma, confusion and dizziness, diarrhea, urinary tract infections, lymphadenopathy, and frequent hospitalizations.

Lesson 6—Inflammation

1. All five patients have developed an acute inflammatory response. The causes of these responses are as follows:
   - Andrea Wang—trauma
   - David Ruskin—trauma
   - Carmen Gonzales—microorganisms
   - Sally Begay—microorganisms
   - Ira Bradley—immune defect, trauma

2. Cellular injury causes mast cell degranulation, activation of the plasma systems (clotting, complement, and kinin), and release of cellular components. This causes vasodilation (redness and heat), vascular permeability (edema), cellular infiltration (pus), thrombosis (clots), and stimulation of nerve endings (pain).

3. Complement system, clotting system, and kinin system

4. Granulocytes and macrophage/monocytes

5. Sally Begay and Ira Bradley

6. Sally Begay:
   - Saturday—monos = 5%, indicating systemic inflammation
   - Tuesday—monos = 3%, indicating normal levels
   Ira Bradley:
   - Sunday—monos = 7.8%, indicating inflammation
   - Tuesday—monos = 5.8%, indicating inflammation, but some improvement

7. Fever, leukocytosis (transient increase in circulating lymphocytes), and increase in circulating plasma proteins

8. Ira Bradley has a fever (100.2° F). His monocyte count is elevated on Sunday (7.8%) and on Tuesday (5.8%).

   Sally Begay has a fever (100.1° F). Her white blood cell count on Saturday is 32.9 and on Tuesday it is 15.7. Her monocyte count is 5% on Saturday and returns to normal (3%) on Tuesday.

9. His ability to mount an effective immune response will be decreased, or he may be incapable of mounting an effective response.

10. Andrea Wang—trauma
    David Ruskin—trauma
    Ira Bradley—trauma
    Carmen Gonzales—microorganisms

11. The local manifestations of inflammation are swelling, pain, heat, redness, and exudate.

12. Andrea Wang—pain
    David Ruskin—acute pain
    Ira Bradley—pain
    Carmen Gonzales—swelling, pain, skin discoloration, and purulent exudate

13. David Ruskin, because he is African-American

14. Keloid formation is caused by an imbalance between collagen synthesis and collagen lysis, in which synthesis is increased and lysis is decreased. A keloid is a raised scar that extends beyond the original boundaries of the wound. It invades surrounding tissue and is likely to recur after surgical removal. A familial tendency to keloid formation has been observed, with greater incidence in blacks than whites.

Lesson 7—Infection and Alterations in Immunity and Inflammation

1. Hantavirus infection

2. Bacterial pneumonia

3. Bacterial survival and growth depend on the effectiveness of the body's defense mechanisms and on the bacterium's ability to resist these defenses. Many pathogens have devised ways of preventing destruction by the inflammatory and immune systems, such as thick capsules. Some pathogens proliferate at rates that surpass the rate of development of the immune system as protective response. Others survive and proliferate in the body by pro-

ducing exotoxins and endotoxins that injure cells and tissues. Some bacteria alter antigens, initiating self-destructive (autoimmune) reactions. Others produce substances that immuno-logically look like host proteins and cause the body to produce an autoimmune reaction against the antigen in normal tissues.

Viruses proliferate within cells by taking over the metabolic machinery for host cells and using it for their own survival and replication. Viruses do not produce exotoxins or endotoxins. Viral pathogens bypass many defense mechanisms by developing intracellu-larly, thus hiding within cells and away from normal inflammatory or immune responses. In many cases, however, because viral agents must spread from cell to cell, the developing immune response eventually cures the infection, so the disease is usually self-limiting. On the other hand, viruses can rapidly produce irreversible and lethal injury to highly suscepti-ble cells in an immunocompromised host. If a symbiotic relationship is maintained between the host cell and the virus, persistent unapparent infection may result. Cell injury does not occur, and the virus persists until it is activated to replicate. Immunity may protect the indi-vidual from an acute exacerbation only, or it may be sufficiently strong to prevent disease.

4. She has a fever, the most common symptom of infection, and an elevated white blood cell count.

5. Erythromycin and ceftizoxime, which are are both antibiotics used to treat bacterial infec-tion.

6. AIDS is caused by the human immunodeficiency virus (HIV).

7. The development of vaccines against HIV has been frustrating because of the large number of changing antigens expressed on the viral surface. Thus the virus can change and adapt to attempts to destroy it and survive.

8. Homosexual and bisexual men; intravenous drug abusers; heterosexual partners of those infected with HIV; recipients of infected blood, blood products, or semen (artificial insemi-nation); fetuses or newborns of infected mothers; and health care workers who come in con-tact with contaminated blood.

9. No, he does not.

10. The HIV virus, a retrovirus carrying genetic information in RNA rather than DNA, causes AIDS. Retroviruses infect cells by binding to the surface of a target cell through a receptor and inserting their RNA into the target cell. Through the use of a viral enzyme, reverse tran-scriptase, the viral RNA is converted to DNA and inserted into the infected cell's genetic material. If the cell is activated, viral proliferation may occur, resulting in the lysis and death of the infected cell. If, however, the cell remains relatively dormant, the viral genetic material is integrated into the infected cell's DNA, may remain latent for years, and proba-bly is present for the life of the individual. CD4 is an antigen on the surface of T helper cells that acts as the primary receptor for HIV. CD4 is known to be necessary, but not sufficient, for HIV fusion with, and entry into, human cells.

Recently, another membrane protein, fusin, was identified as a cofactor. Fusin, however, has been identified in only a few strains of HIV and not in the wide variety that exist in the community. The virus infects primarily CD4-positive T helper lymphocytes but may infect various other cells of the central nervous system that also express the CD2 antigen. Once activated, the virus causes the destruction of the CD4-positive cells, causing a marked decrease in CD4 cells. CD4 depletion has a profound effect on the immune system—most notably, a severely diminished response to a wide array of infectious pathogens and malig-nant tumors. The precise destruction of CD4-positive cells remains unknown, but most of the cells undergoing cellular death do not appear to be infected with HIV.

11. Lymphadenopathy, weight loss, recurrent fevers, neuralgic abnormalities (confusion and dizziness), recurrent pulmonary infiltrates, and evidence of opportunistic infections (PCP, candidiasis, and Kaposi's sarcoma).

12. Medications used to help treat his HIV infection include trimethoprim and sulfamethoxazole, delavirdine myselate, saquinovir, fluconazole, and alitretinoin gel.

Lesson 8—Stress and Disease

1. The three stages of the general adaptation syndrome are the alarm stage, the stage of resistance or adaptation, and the stage of exhaustion.

2. Andrea Wang, David Ruskin, and Carmen Gonzales are in the resistance or adaptation stage. Sally Begay is in the stage of resistance or adaptation, but because of her suspected decreased immunity, she may be approaching the state of exhaustion. Ira Bradley is in the stage of exhaustion.

3. Ira Bradley's stressors include the downward trajectory of his terminal disease process, frequent infections, malnutrition, dehydration, immobility, inability to work, and frequent hospitalizations. Family stressors include overwhelmed family coping mechanisms, resulting in a disintegrating family structure, isolation, loss of support group and friends, financial problems, and uncertainty about the future.

4. As Ira Bradley's disease process progresses, stressors for him and his family are increasing and their coping resources are depleted. Social support systems, which are critical when coping with end-of-life issues, are absent. Ira Bradley will continue his downward spiral toward death, and his wife and children are at major risk for physical illness from their high stress levels.

5. David Ruskin has no stress-related diseases at present, but he has a family history of coronary artery disease and type 2 diabetes mellitus, so he is at risk for those. Andrea Wang has none at present, but she has a family history of hypertension, diabetes, and stroke; therefore she is at risk for those diseases. Carmen Gonzales has congestive heart failure (a complication of coronary artery disease), mild hypertension, and type 2 diabetes mellitus. Sally Begay has coronary artery disease and mild hypertension. Ira Bradley has depression.

6. With aging, certain neurohormonal and immune alterations, as well as tissue and cellular changes, sometimes develop; these stress-age syndrome changes include:
   - Alterations in the excitability of structures of the limbic system and hypothalamus
   - Rise of the blood concentrations of catecholamines, antidiuretic hormone, adrenocorticotropic hormone, and cortisol
   - Decrease in testosterone, thyroxine, and other hormones
   - Alterations of opioid peptides
   - Immunodepression
   - Alterations in lipoproteins
   - Hypercoagulation of the blood
   - Free radical damage to cells

   Some of the alterations are adaptational, whereas others are potentially damaging. These stress-related alterations of aging can influence the course of developing stress reactions and lower adaptive reserve and coping.

Lesson 9—Biology of Cancer

1. Ira Bradley has Kaposi's sarcoma, a rare form of blood vessel cancer in the skin.

2. Human immunodeficiency viral infection

3. HIV is a retrovirus that has been implicated as causing cancers. HIV is the causative agent of AIDS, a disease associated with a high incidence of B cell lymphoma and Kaposi's sarcoma. It appears, however, that HIV is not directly involved in the development of human cancers.

4. Oncogenic viruses are divided into two major groups according to nucleic acid content of the viral particle—DNA or RNA. The three main types of DNA oncogenic viruses are papovaviruses, adenoviruses, and herpesviruses. DNA viruses penetrate host cells by the action of their coat proteins. Inside the cell the viral DNA is uncoated and enters the cell's nucleus, where it sets up replication. Major cancers from these viruses are cancer of the cervix and hepatocellular carcinoma.

   RNA oncogenic viruses are retroviruses containing reverse transcriptase, the enzyme required for successful infection. Once the viral genome has been transcribed to viral DNA, it can be integrated into the host's DNA, where it is transcribed and replicated. The major cancer caused by these viruses in humans is human T leukemia/lymphoma.

5. HIV is an RNA virus (retrovirus); however it does not directly cause cancer in humans.

6. Tumor growth or rejection depends on complex interactions between cancer cells and the immune system of their host. Many immunologic protective mechanisms that cause tumor lysis have been identified. For certain types of neoplasia there is an increased risk of 2% to 20% for developing cancer in individuals who are immunosuppressed. Immunologic suppression also enhances the growth and recurrence of tumors in individuals with preexisting cancers.

Lesson 10—Tumor Invasion and Metastasis

1. On his left thigh

2. Invasion, or local spread, is a prerequisite for metastasis and is the first step in the metastatic process. In its earliest stages, local invasion may occur as a function of direct tumor extension. Eventually, however, cells or clumps of cells become detached from the primary tumor and invade the surrounding interstitial spaces. Possible mechanisms thought to be important in local invasion include cellular multiplication, mechanical pressure, release of lytic enzymes, decreased cell-to-cell adhesion, and increased motility of individual tumor cells. These mechanisms are not mutually exclusive, and it is likely that in a given tumor, any combination of the five may be involved.

3. Metastasis, the spread of cancer from a primary site of origin to a distant site, is the life-threatening characteristic of malignancy. Local invasion is a condition of metastasis. Methods exist for successfully eradicating primary tumors. The real challenge for reducing cancer mortality is controlling metastasis, because removal of the primary tumor does not affect the proliferating growth at other sites. Often the primary tumor is not even diagnosed before secondary spread occurs. Three basic methods for metastasis exist—direct or continuous extension, lymphatic spread, and bloodstream dissemination. These mechanisms are not mutually exclusive. Tumor cell spread or dissemination through one mechanism often facilitates metastasis through other mechanisms, because tumor cells move through numerous microscopic anatomic connections.

4. No. Ira Bradley has none of these signs and symptoms.

5. Pain, fatigue, cachexia, anemia, leukopenia, thrombocytopenia, and infection

6. Ira Bradley manifests pain, fatigue, cachexia, anemia, and infection.

7. No. He is not taking any of these chemotherapeutic drugs.

Lesson 11—Pain, Temperature Regulation, Sleep, and Sensory Function

1. All five patients are experiencing some kind of pain:
   - Sally Begay has chest pain when she coughs.
   - Carmen Gonzales has pain in her wound.
   - Ira Bradley has a headache and pain with swallowing.
   - Andrea Wang has pain in the back, shoulders, and arms.
   - David Ruskin has a headache and pain in his fractured arm.

2. Three systems interact to produce pain. They are the sensory/discriminative system, the motivational/affective system, and the cognitive/evaluative system.
   - The sensory/discriminative system processes information about the strength, intensity, and temporal and spatial aspects of pain. These sensations are mediated through afferent nerve fibers, the spinal cord, the brain stem, and the higher brain centers, and they result in prompt withdrawal from the painful stimulus.
   - The motivational/affective system determines the individual's conditioned or learned approach/avoidance behaviors. These behaviors are mediated through the interaction of the recticular formation, limbic system, and brain stem.
   - The cognitive/evaluative system overlies the individual's learned behavior concerning the experience of pain. The individual's interpretation of appropriate pain behavior is learned in several ways, including them the cultural preferences, male and female roles, and experience. The influence of the cognitive/evaluative system may block, modulate, or enhance the perception of pain.

3. Studies on pain perception in older adults have yielded conflicting evidence. Some studies show an increase in the pain threshold with aging; others show no change. The varied results are probably a function of independent variation in the sensory/discriminative, motivational/affective, and cognitive/evaluative components of the pain experience. In general, studies confirm that an increase in the pain threshold occurs in some older adults. This change probably is caused by peripheral neuropathies and changes in the thickness of the skin. A decrease in pain tolerance is also evident in aging persons, and women appear to be more sensitive to pain than are men.

4. Physiologic responses to acute pain include increased heart rate, elevated blood pressure, pallor or flushing, dilated pupils, diaphoresis, elevated blood sugar levels, decreased gastric secretions and intestinal motility, decreased blood flow to the viscera and skin, and occasional nausea.

5. David Ruskin complains of extreme pain in his right arm, but he has no physiologic responses noted.
   Andrea Wang has flushed and decreased intestinal motility (hypoactive bowel sounds).
   Carmen Gonzales is experiencing nausea, and her heart rate and blood pressure are elevated.
   Ira Bradley has pain in his esophagus and head, but he has no physiologic responses noted.
   Sally Begay has an increased heart rate, an elevated blood pressure, and nausea.

6. Carmen Gonzales has fever because of her leg infection.
   Sally Begay has fever because of her pneumonia.
   Ira Bradley has fever because of his dehydration and infection.

7. Simple raising of the body temperature kills many microorganisms and has adverse effects on the growth and replication of others. Higher body temperatures decrease serum levels of iron, zinc, and copper, all of which are needed for bacterial replication. The body switches from burning glucose to a metabolism based on lipolysis and proteolysis, thus depriving bacteria of a food source. Anorexia and somnolence reduce the demand for muscle glucose. Increased temperature also causes lysosomal breakdown and autodestruction of cells, thus preventing viral replication in infected cells. Acute-phase proteins produced by the liver bind cations necessary for bacterial reproduction. Heat increases lymphocytic transforma-

tion and motility of polymorphonuclear neutrophils, thus facilitating the immune response. Phagocytosis is enhanced, and production of antiviral interferon may be augmented.

8. David Ruskin and Andrea Wang are at risk for malignant hyperthermia, a potentially lethal complication of a rare inherited muscle disorder. The condition is precipitated by the administration of volatile anesthetics and neuromuscular blocking agents. About 1 in 200 individuals may be at risk for this disorder. Malignant hyperthermia is caused by either increased calcium release or decreased calcium uptake with muscular contraction. This allows intracellular calcium levels to rise, producing sustained, uncoordinated muscle contractions, which in turn increase muscle work, oxygen consumption, and lactic acid production. As a result of these contractions, acidosis develops and temperature rises (as quickly at 1° C every 5 minutes); approximately 20% of those who develop malignant hyperthermia do not survive. Malignant hyperthermia occurs most often in children and young adults immediately after the induction of anesthesia. Sympathetic responses and acidosis produce tachycardia and cardiac dysrhythmias, followed by hypotension, decreased cardiac output, and, eventually, cardiac arrest. Increasing temperature, acidosis, hyperkalemia, and hypoxia produce coma-like symptoms in the CNS, including unconsciousness, absent reflexes, fixed pupils, apnea, and sometimes, flat electroencephalogram. Oliguria and anuria are common, probably resulting from shock, ischemia, and low cardiac output. Treatment includes withdrawal of the provoking agents and administration of dantrolene sodium, a skeletal relaxant that inhibits calcium release during muscle contraction. Pronestyl is used to treat cardiac dysrhythmias. Sodium bicarbonate also may be used. Body temperature is decreased through use of ice bags, cooling blankets, and iced saline lavage.

9. Carmen Gonzales and Ira Bradley

10. With aging, total sleep time is decreased, and the older individual takes longer to fall asleep. Older adults awaken earlier in the morning and more frequently during the night. Total REM stage and stage II time is unchanged, but stage IV sleep decreases by 15% to 30%. On EEG results, the spindle indicating stage II sleep is less well formed. These changes in the older adult's sleep pattern may be associated with changes in lifestyle, physical ailments, lack of daily routine, desynchronization of circadian rhythm, and use of sedatives. Growth hormones and cortisol are diminished in older adults and may affect sleep patterns. The alteration in sleep pattern typically appears about 10 years later in women than in men. Older adults are less able than younger individuals to tolerate sleep deprivation.

11. Normal sensory changes in older adults include the following:
Eyes
- Increase in astigmatism from thicker less curved lens
- Arcus senilis formation
- Decrease in size and volume of the anterior chamber
- Increased lens opacity, which can lead to cataracts
- Increased firmness and reduced elasticity of the lens, causing presbyopia
- Reduced pupil diameter and atrophy of radial dilation muscles
- In the retina, a reduction of number of rods at periphery and a general loss of rods and associated nerve cells
Ears
- Degeneration of cochlear hair cells, causing inability to hear high-frequency sounds and understand speech
- Loss of auditory neurons in spiral ganglia of the organ of Conti, causing inability to hear high-frequency sounds and understand speech
- Degeneration of basilar conductive membrane of cochlea, causing inability to hear at all frequencies
- Decreased vascularity of cochlea, resulting in equal hearing loss at all frequencies and inability to disseminate localization of sound
- Loss of cortical auditory neurons, resulting in equal hearing loss at all frequencies and inability to disseminate localization of sound

Nose
- Decline in sensitivity to odors
- Degeneration of sense of smell

Mouth
- Decline in taste sensation
- Decreased salivary gland secretion

12. No, she does not.

Lesson 12—Concepts of Neurologic Dysfunction

1. David Ruskin and Ira Bradley

2. Three pathophysiologic mechanisms probably underlie the development of acute confusional states associated with delirium. These are:
   - Injury to the nervous tissue
   - Action of toxin or chemical agents on neuronal cells
   - Inhibition of overactivity of a previously depressed brain center

   Destructive injuries directly affect the nervous tissues and disturb the function of the neurons. In states of intoxication, the direct action of toxins or chemicals on neuronal cells produces dysfunction of the involved cells. In states of withdrawal, the lower brain centers are overactive after the depressant action of the drug wears off; this overactivity accounts for the development of the acute confusional state.

3. Difficulty in concentration, restlessness, irritability, tremulousness, insomnia, and poor appetite

4. Ira Bradley's clinical manifestations are impaired attention, disorientation, and poor appetite. David Ruskin's clinical manifestation is disorientation.

5. Both are at risk for cerebral edema, which if untreated, will lead to increased intracranial pressure and herniation syndromes.

6. The four types of cerebral edema are vasogenic, cytotoxic (metabolic), ischemic, and interstitial.
   - Vasogenic edema is clinically the most important type. It is caused by the increased permeability of the capillary endothelium of the brain after injury to the vascular structure. The result is a disruption in the blood-brain barrier. Plasma proteins leak into the extracellular spaces, drawing water to them, and the water content of the brain parenchyma increases. Vasogenic edema starts in the area of injury and spreads with preferential accumulation in the white matter of the ipsilateral side because the parallel myelinated fibers separate more easily. Edema then promotes further edema because of ischemia from increasing pressure.
   - In cytotoxic (metabolic) edema, toxic factors directly affect the cellular elements of the brain parenchyma, causing failure of the active transport systems. The cells lose their potassium and gain larger amounts of sodium. Water follows by osmosis into the cell, so that the cells swell. Cytotoxic edema occurs principally in the gray matter and may increase vasogenic edema.
   - Ischemic edema follows cerebral infarction and has components of both vasogenic and cytotoxic edema.
   - Interstitial edema is seen most often with noncommunicating hydrocephalus and is caused by an over-accumulation of CSF.

   David Ruskin is at risk for vasogenic edema.

7. Clinical manifestations of vasogenic edema include focal neurologic deficits, disturbances of consciousness, and severe increase in intracranial pressure. Vasogenic edema resolves by slow diffusion.

8. No. Neither of these patients exhibits any clinic manifestations of cerebral edema.

9. Yes. Andrea Wang has paralysis/paresis with upper motor neuron syndrome. Paraparesis/paraplegia refers to paresis/paralysis of the lower extremities. Lower cord damage results in paraparesis/paraplegia. Her spinal cord injury is incomplete, meaning that she maintains some function.

Lesson 13—Alterations of Neurologic Function

1. David Ruskin and Ira Bradley

2. Transportation-related events (48%) and falls cause most traumatic brain injuries. Sports-related events and violence also account for a portion of craniocerebral traumatic brain injury.

3. David Ruskin's head trauma was caused by a fall during a sports-related event (riding his bicycle). Ira Bradley's head trauma was caused by a fall.

4. Focal brain injury refers to specific grossly observable brain lesions—cortical contusion, epidural hemorrhage, subdural hematoma, and intracerebral hematoma. The force of impact (translational acceleration) typically produces contusions from direct contact (as well as injury to the vault, vessels, and supporting structures), which in turn produce epidural hemorrhage and subdural and intracerebral hematomas. Damage results from compression of the skull at the point of impact and rebound effect. Contusions and bleeding occur because of small tears in blood vessels resulting from these forces. The severity of the contusion is associated with the amount of energy transmitted by the skull to underlying brain tissue. In addition, the smaller the area of impact, the greater the severity of injury because the force is concentrated into a smaller area. The focal injury may be coup or contrecoup. Brain edema forms around and in the damaged neural tissues, contributing to the increasing intracranial pressure. Within the contused areas are infarctions and necrosis, multiple hemorrhages, and edema. The tissue has a pulpy quality. The maximum effects of injury related to contusion, bleeding, and edema peak 18 to 36 hours after severe head injury.

5. David Ruskin had immediate loss of consciousness when the event occurred. He was not oriented to time, place, or situation upon arrival to the emergency department.

6. Ira Bradley had no documented loss of consciousness at the time of the event. He was disoriented upon arrival to the emergency department.

7. Andrea Wang

8. Spinal cord injuries most commonly occur because of vertebral injuries, which are a result of acceleration, deceleration, or deformation forces, most frequently applied at a distance. These forces injure the vertebral or neural tissues by compressing the tissues, pulling or exerting a traction (tension) on the tissues, or shearing tissues so that they slide into one another. These forces may be exerted on the vertebral and neural tissues by hyperextension, hyperflexion, vertical compression, or rotation of the spine. The bones, ligaments, and joints of the vertebral column may be damaged. The vertebral column may incur fracture and often compression of one or more elements, dislocation of its elements, or both fracture and dislocation. Vertebral injuries can be classified as simple fracture (a single break, usually affecting transverse or spinous processes), compressed or wedged vertebral fracture (vertebral body compressed anteriorly), comminuted (burst) fracture (vertebral body shattered into several fragments), or dislocation. Vertebral injuries occur mostly at vertebrae C1 to C2, C4 to C7, and T1 to L2 because these are the most mobile portions of the vertebral column. The cord occupies most of the vertebral canal in the cervical and lumbar regions. The size makes the cord in these areas more easily injured. Noncontiguous vertebral injuries are not uncommon.

Within a few minutes after injury, microscopic hemorrhages appear in the central gray matter and pia arachnoid; these hemorrhages increase in size within 2 hours. Edema in the white matter occurs, impairing the microcirculation of the cord. Within 4 hours, numerous swollen axis cylinders develop. Reduced vascular perfusion and development of ischemic areas follow localized hemorrhaging and edema. Oxygen tension in the tissue at the injury site is decreased. The microscopic hemorrhages and edema are maximal at the level of injury and for two cord segments above and below it. Cellular and subcellular alterations and tissue necrosis occur. Chemical and metabolic changes in spinal cord tissue include release of toxic excitatory amino acids, accumulation of endogenous opiates, lipid hydrolysis with production of active metabolites, and local free radical release. These changes may produce further ischemia, vascular damage, and necrosis of tissues (autodestruction). Cord swelling increases the individual's degree of dysfunction, so that it becomes difficult to distinguish the functions that are lost from those that are only temporarily impaired. Within the first few days of injury, progressive axonal changes occur and necrotic zones develop. Progressive cavitation and coagulation necrosis at the site of injury are termed *posttraumatic infarction*. Circulation to the white matter tracts of the spinal cord returns to normal in about 24 hours, but gray matter circulation remains altered. The traumatized cord is replaced by acellular collagenous tissue, usually in 3 to 4 weeks. Meninges thicken as part of the scarring process.

9. Spinal shock is characterized by complete loss of reflex function in all segments below the level of the lesion. This condition involves all skeletal muscles, bladder, bowel, sexual function, and autonomic control. Severe impairment below the level of the lesion is obvious; it includes paralysis and flaccidity of muscles, absence of sensation, loss of bladder and rectal control, transient drop in blood pressure, and poor venous circulation. The condition also results in disturbed thermal control because the sympathetic nervous system is damaged. This damage causes faulty control of sweating and radiation through capillary dilation. The hypothalmic center cannot regulate body heat through vasoconstriction and increased metabolism; therefore the individual assumes the temperature of the air. Spinal shock may last from 7 to 20 days after onset; it may persist for as short a time as a few days or as long as 3 months.

10. Andrea Wang has no sensation below the nipple line. Her skin is flushed and warm to touch, indicating injury to the sympathetic nervous system. She has flaccid paralysis below the level of injury, her bowel sounds are hypoactive, her rectal tone is diminished, and her bladder is distended.

11. Indications that spinal shock is terminating include the reappearance of reflex activity, hyperreflexia, spasticity, and reflex emptying of the bladder.

12. Her deep tendon reflexes in her lower extremities are noted to be hyperactive during physical examination.

13. Autonomic hyperreflexia (dysreflexia)

14. Autonomic hyperreflexia (dysreflexia) is a syndrome that may occur at any time after spinal shock resolves. The syndrome is associated with a massive, uncompensated cardiovascular response to stimulation of the sympathetic nervous system. The condition is life-threatening and requires immediate treatment. Individuals most likely to be affected have lesions at the T6 level or above. It is characterized by paroxysmal hypertension (up to 300 mm Hg systolic), a pounding headache, blurred vision, sweating above the level of the lesion with flushing of the skin, nasal congestion, nausea, piloerection caused by pilomotor spasm, and bradycardia (often dropping to 30 to 40 beats per minute). The symptoms may develop singly or in combination. The pathophysiology of hyperreflexia involves the stimulation of sensory receptors below the level of the cord lesion. The intact autonomic nervous system reflexively responds with an arteriolar spasm that increases blood pressure. Baroreceptors in the cerebral vessels, the carotid sinus, and the aorta sense the hypertension and stimulate the

parasympathetic system. The heart rate decreases, but the visceral and peripheral vessels do not dilate because efferent impulses cannot pass through the cord.

15. She exhibits hypertension, splitting headache, blurred vision, sweating and flushing above the level of the lesion, nasal congestion, nausea, and bradycardia.

16. The most common cause is a distended bladder or rectum, but any sensory stimulation can elicit autonomic hyperreflexia.

17. A distended bladder

Lesson 14—Neurobiology of Schizophrenia, Mood Disorders, and Anxiety Disorders

1. Ira Bradley

2. Depression is the most common mood disorder. There is a strong genetic basis for development of depression; however environmental factors are thought to have a strong potentiating effect. The pathophysiology of depression is not completely understood. In one theory, depression is hypothesized to occur following a deficit of brain norepinephrine or serotonin. Another theory hypothesizes that an abnormality in the hypothalmic-pituitary-adrenal systems causes depression. A third theory postulates that neuroanatomic and functional abnormalities contribute to depression.

3. Clinical manifestations of depression include the following:
   - Depressed mood
   - Loss of interests and pleasure
   - Irritability
   - Sadness
   - Decrease or increase in appetite
   - Insomnia
   - Psychomotor agitation or retardation
   - Fatigue
   - Feelings of worthlessness
   - Excessive guilt
   - Poor concentration
   - Suicidal thoughts

4. Decreased appetite and insomnia

5. Depression is treated with medication (MAO inhibitors, tricyclic antidepressants, and SSRIs). Those who do not respond may receive electroconvulsive therapy. Lithium is sometimes used in long-term maintenance to prevent further relapses.

6. The primary etiology of posttraumatic stress disorder is exposure to a major stressor and may involve several neural structures, including the locus ceruleus, the hippocampus and the amygdala. The amygdala may play an especially important role in posttraumatic stress disorder because of its involvement in the acquisition and extinction of learned fear responses. Furthermore, it has diverse connections to sensory cortical regions where memories may be stored. Activation of the amygdala may lead to the recollection of traumatic memories. Several neurochemical systems also may play a role in the development of posttraumatic stress disorder. These neurotransmitter systems include norepinepherine, dopamine, opiate, and corticotropin-releasing factors. Secretion or elevated concentrations of these neurotransmitters frequently occur during stressful conditions.

7. Persons with a history of psychiatric disorders (major depression, panic disorder) or those who lack strong social support are most likely to develop posttraumatic stress disorder.

8. No. She has no history of psychiatric disorder and has strong social supports.

9. Difficulty sleeping, irritability, lack of concentration, hypervigilance, and exaggerated startle response

10. No

11. It is treated with psychotherapy and antidepressant medication.

Lesson 15—Alterations of Hormonal Regulation

1. Type 2 diabetes mellitus

2. The endocrine pancreas

3. The diagnosis of diabetes is based on one of the following:
   - More than one fasting plasma glucose level greater than or equal to 126 mg/dl.
   - Plasma glucose value (in the 2-hour sample of the standard oral glucose tolerance test) of greater than or equal to 200 mg/dl, confirmed on subsequent day
   - Causal plasma glucose level (any time of day without regard to time since last meal) greater than 200 mg/dl, combined with classic symptoms of polydipsia, polyphagia, and polyuria

4. The cause of type 2 DM is unknown, and genetics of this form are complex and not clearly defined. Type 2 DM affects people primarily after the age of 40, many of whom are obese. Cellular response to the effect of insulin is a major factor and is heightened by obesity, inactivity, illnesses, medications, and age. Abnormal glucagon secretion has also been demonstrated. A significant body of evidence has accumulated indicating that a defect in insulin secretion can lead to insulin resistance and vice versa. Once type 2 DM has become established, it is impossible to determine in any given individual whether the primary defect originated in the beta cell or in peripheral or hepatic tissues. Eventually the beta cell responsiveness to the glucose stimulus diminishes and hyperglycemia supervenes. Most individuals with type 2 DM are hyperinsulinemic at the time of diagnosis but have a relative deficiency of insulin. The islet dysfunction may be caused by a decrease in beta cell mass, abnormal function of the beta cells, or some combination. A decrease in the weight and number of beta cells generally occurs in type 2 DM, but the cause is unclear. The decrease in beta cells may be the result of progressive deterioration over time. To confuse the issue further, the ratio of alpha cells to beta cells may be completely normal, and most individuals have plasma and pancreatic insulin levels that are not decreased.

5.
Day	Time	Level
Sunday	2000	267 mg/dl
Tuesday	0800	272 mg/dl
Tuesday	2000	167 mg/dl

6. All her levels are elevated, but they are decreasing over time.

7.
Day	Time	Level
Sunday	2400	268 mg/dl
Monday	0800	250 mg/dl
Monday	2000	185 mg/dl
Monday	2400	190 mg/dl
Tuesday	2000	160 mg/dl
Tuesday	2400	160 mg/dl
Wednesday	0800	145 mg/dl
Wednesday	1200	160 mg/dl
Wednesday	1600	155 mg/dl

Wednesday	2000	160 mg/dl
Thursday	1600	145 mg/dl
Thursday	2000	145 mg/dl
Thursday	2400	142 mg/dl
Friday	0800	142 mg/dl

8. All her values are elevated, but the trend is a decrease over time.

9. Age greater than 40 years and obesity

10. Both—she is 56 years of age and she is obese (5 feet 2 inches and 170 pounds).

11. She is over 40, female, in a high-risk ethnic group (Hispanic), of lower economic status (fixed income), and obese.

12. Obesity, dyslipidemia, hyperinsulinemia, and hypertension

13. Obesity and hypertension

14. Nonspecific symptoms of type 2 DM:
    * Recurrent infections—boils, carbuncles, skin infections
    * Prolonged wound healing
    * Genital pruritis
    * Visual changes
    * Paresthesias
    * Fatigue

15. Fatigue, recurrent infections, and visual changes (blurring)

16. Weight loss, exercise, and a diet low in fat and carbohydrates

17. Hypoglycemia and hyperosmolar, hyperglycemic, nonketotic syndrome

18. Chronic complications of diabetes mellitus:
    * Diabetic neuropathies
    * Microvascular disease—retinopathy, diabetic nephropathy
    * Macrovascular disease—coronary artery disease, stroke, peripheral vascular disease
    * Infection

19. Carmen Gonzales exhibits the following chronic complications:
    * Retinopathy—In the Review of Systems section of the Physical & History, she complains of blurred vision.
    * Coronary artery disease—Her previous medical history lists a diagnosis of coronary artery disease.
    * Peripheral vascular disease—In her Emergency Department Record, she is noted to have faint pulses below the knees and delayed capillary refill.
    * Infection—She has been admitted for an infected wound on her leg.

Lesson 16—Alterations of the Reproductive Systems

1. Carmen Gonzales is at risk for vaginitis. She has type 2 diabetes mellitus, which increases the glycogen content of vaginal secretions. This alters the bacteriocidal nature of the secretions, predisposing her to vaginal infections.

2. No, but the genital examination on the Physical & History was deferred.

3. Yes, because she is not having preventative screening and the rate of cervical cancer has recently increased in women over 50 years of age.

4. Premalignant lesions occur 10 to 12 years before the development of invasive carcinoma. The progressive changes of cervical cells are classified on a continuum from cervical intraepithelial neoplasia, to cervical carcinoma in situ to invasive carcinoma. Cervical intraepithelial neoplasia or cervical dysplasia, is replacement of some epithelial cells by atypical, neoplastic cells and is graded as mild, moderate, severe, or carcinoma in situ. Women with mild neoplasia have a 15% chance of developing cancer; severe, 75%. Carcinoma in situ is most likely to develop in the transformation zone, where columnar epithelium of the cervical lining meets the squamous epithelium of the outer cervix and vagina. It is generally a precursor to invasive carcinoma of the cervix. Invasive carcinoma of the cervix consists of direct invasion into adjacent tissues and metastasis through the lymphatics.

5. Early cervical cancer is asymptomatic.

6. It is diagnosed through regular cytology screening by Pap smear.

7. She is concerned about her level of sexual function (what she will be able to do).

8. It is difficult to tell since her lesion is incomplete and she may regain more function. In the worst-case scenario, she will have reflex sexual response, decreased sensation and lubrication, and altered arousal. Orgasmic sensations may be diffused in general or to specific body parts.

9. Vascular disorders, endocrine disorders, neurologic disorders, chronic disease, genitourinary disorders, psychologic disorders, and iatrogenic factors such as drugs and surgery.

10. Chronic disease in the terminal stages, psychologic problems, and frequent urinary tract infections

Lesson 17—Sexually Transmitted Infections

1. Syphilis facilitates the transmission of HIV infection and seems to contribute to HIV transmission in those parts of the United States where incidence of both infections are high.

2. Low-grade fever, malaise, sore throat, hoarseness, anorexia, generalized adenopathy, headache, joint pain, and skin or mucous membrane lesions or rashes. Also, pruritis, alopecia, anemia, leukocytosis, increased sedimentation rate, hepatitis, transitory proteinuria, arthritis, ECG changes, and CNS symptoms.

3. Yes. Ira Bradley exhibits low-grade fever, malaise, sore throat, hoarseness, anorexia, headache, skin and mucous membrane lesions, anemia, leukocytosis, and CNS symptoms.

4. VDRL and RPR

5. No

6. Molluscum contagiosum

7. White or flesh-colored, round or oval, domed-shaped papules

8. Individuals with AIDS may develop extensive lesions over the face, neck, and genital regions.

9. No

10. Cytomegalovirus (CMV)

11. CMV can be a devastating, life-threatening illness.

12. No

Lesson 18—Alterations of Erythrocyte Function

1. Hematocrit—40% to 50%
   Hemoglobin—13.5 to 18.0 g/dl

2. Carmen Gonzales, Sally Begay, and Ira Bradley

3. Carmen Gonzales has a low hematocrit and hemoglobin and a normal red blood cell count and mean corpuscular volume, consistent with anemia of chronic inflammation.
   Carmen Gonzales has a low hematocrit and hemoglobin and a normal red blood cell count and mean corpuscular volume, consistent with anemia of chronic inflammation.
   Ira Bradley has low hematocrit, hemoglobin, red blood cell count, and mean corpuscular volume, consistent with iron deficiency anemia.

4. **Anemia of chronic inflammation:** Presence of chronic inflammation; otherwise may be asymptomatic.
   Iron deficiency anemia: Fatigue; weakness; shortness of breath; pale earlobes, palms, and conjunctiva; brittle, thin, coarsely ridged, and concave nails; sore, red, burning tongue; angular stomatitis; dysphagia; gastritis; neuromuscular changes; irritability; headache; numbness; tingling; vasomotor disturbances; memory loss; mental confusion; and disorientation.

5. Carmen Gonzales has a chronic inflammatory response with her infected leg.
   Sally Begay has a chronic inflammatory response with her chronic bronchitis.
   Ira Bradley has fatigue, weakness, shortness of breath, mental confusion, disorientation, and dysphagia.

Lesson 19—Alterations of Leukocyte, Lymphoid, and Hemostatic Function

1.

Lab Test	Normal Counts	Carmen Gonzales	Sally Begay
WBC	5,000–10,000 mm^3	18,200 mm^3	32,900 mm^3
Neutrophils	57%–67%	70% segs 20% bands	24% segs 1% bands
Lymphocytes	25%–33%	14%	67%
Monocytes	3%–7%	9%	5%
Eosinophils	1%–4%	4%	0%
Basophils	0%–0.75%	0%	1%

2. Both Carmen Gonzales and Sally Begay have leukocytosis.

3. Segs and bands

4. Sally Begay—infection

5. Carmen Gonzales—inflammation, infection, and tissue necrosis

6. Carmen Gonzales—decreased immunity, debilitating illness such as osteomyelitis

7. Sally Begay—acute infection (pneumonia)

8. Carmen Gonzales—bacterial infection

9. Carmen Gonzales—inflammation

10. Triad of Virchow is a list of the predisposing factors that promote thrombus formation and includes:
    • Injury to the blood vessel endothelium
    • Abnormalities in blood flow
    • Hypercoagulability of the blood

11. Andrea Wang is at highest risk: major surgery, SCI, limb paralysis, bedrest longer than 1 week.
    Ira Bradley is at risk—malignancy.
    Carmen Gonzales is at risk—congestive heart failure, advanced age, bedrest longer than 1 week.
    Sally Begay may be at risk—symptoms of congestive heart failure.

Lesson 20—Alterations of Cardiovascular Function

1. The lesions progress from endothelial injury to fatty streak to fibrotic plaque to complicated lesion. The oxidation of LDL is an important step in atherosclerosis and results in recruitment of more macrophages to the area, which then engulf the oxidized LDL and penetrate into the intima of the vessel. Macrophages that are full of oxidized LDL are called *foam cells* and are the first pathologic finding in atherogenesis. The next stage in atherogenesis involves the incorporation of fibrous tissue and damaged smooth muscle cells into the area overlying the foam cells, forming a cap called a *fibrous plaque* or *fibroadenoma*. This results in further endothelial dysfunction, necrosis of underlying vessel tissue, and narrowing of the vessel lumen as the lesion protrudes out of the wall. This plaque causes progressive resistance to blood blow and can cause distal ischemia, especially under conditions in which there is an increased demand for perfusion by the affected tissues. As the plaque continues to develop, it can ulcerate or rupture because of mechanical shear forces and continued necrosis of the vessel wall. Platelets aggregate and adhere to the surface of the ruptured plaque, the coagulation cascade is initiated, and a thrombus forms over the lesion that may completely obstruct the lumen of the vessel.

2. Smoking, hypertension, diabetes, turbulent blood flow, increased fibrinogen, autoimmunity, and bacteria and viruses

3. Sally Begay—hypertension
   Carmen Gonzales—hypertension, diabetes

4. Sally Begay—134/76
   Carmen Gonzales—145/84

5. Carmen Gonzales

6. Both Carmen Gonzales and Sally Begay

7. Both Carmen Gonzales and Sally Begay seem to have primary hypertension.

8. Family history of hypertension, advancing age, gender, African-American ethnicity, high dietary sodium intake, glucose intolerance, cigarette smoking, obesity, and heavy alcohol consumption.

9. Carmen Gonzales has advancing age, glucose intolerance, and obesity. Sally Begay has family history of hypertension and possible high sodium intake.

10. Carmen Gonzales does not know the names of her current medications. Sally Begay is taking hydrochlorothiazide, a diuretic.

11. Dietary sodium restriction to 2 g/day, restricted saturated fat intake, calorie adjustment to maintain optimum weight, and development of an exercise plan that promotes endurance and relaxation

12. Carmen Gonzales

13. **Modifiable**
Hypertension
Type 2 diabetes mellitus
Obesity
Sedentary lifestyle

   Nonmodifiable
Advancing age

14. The incidence of CAD in premenopausal women is lower than in men of the same age group. In postmenopausal women the incidence of CAD increases rapidly, and by age 70 the incidence approaches the same rate as that for men.

15. Her CAD will increase more rapidly than it did before menopause.

16. Beginning hormone replacement therapy with estrogen

17. **Stable angina**: classic, exertional angina caused by luminal narrowing and hardening of the arterial walls so that the affected vessels cannot dilate in response to increased myocardial demand associated with physical exertion or emotional stress
Unstable angina: preinfarction angina, acute coronary insufficiency, or crescendo angina and may indicate advanced ischemic heart disease
Variant angina, or Prinzmetal angina: chest pain attributable to transmural ischemia of the myocardium (involves the entire thickness of the myocardial layer)

18. Stable angina

19. | Time | Tissue Changes |
|------|----------------|
| 6–12 hours | No gross changes, subcellular cyanosis with decreased temperature |
| 18–24 hours | Pale to gray-brown, slight pallor from inflammatory response and intercellular enzyme release |
| 2–4 days | Visible necrosis, yellow-brown in the center and hyperemic around the edges |
| 4–10 days | Area soft, with fatty changes in center, regions of hemorrhage in the infarcted area |
| 10–14 days | Weak, fibrotic scar tissue with beginning revascularization |
| 6 weeks | Scarring usually complete |

20. Mild congestive heart failure

21. Both patients have been diagnosed with CHF.

22.

Signs and Symptoms	Sally Begay	Carmen Gonzales
Dyspnea	X	X
Orthopnea		
Cough with frothy sputum		
Fatigue	X	X
Decreased urine output		
Edema		X
Cyanosis		
Rales		X
Hypotension or hypertension	X	X
S_3 gallop		
Pleural effusion		X

23. Elevated systemic venous pressure—seen in Carmen Gonzales as jugular venous distension
Peripheral edema—seen in Carmen Gonzales
Hepatosplenomegaly—seen in Carmen Gonzales as abdominal pain and nausea

Lesson 21—Alterations of Pulmonary Function

1.

Signs and Symptoms	Ira Bradley	Sally Begay
Dyspnea	X	X
Hypoventilation or hyperventilation	X	X
Abnormal breathing patterns		
Cough		X
Hemoptysis		
Cyanosis		
Pain	X	X
Clubbing		
Abnormal sputum		X

2. Chronic bronchitis

3. The most probable cause is air pollution related to farm work since there is no evidence that she has ever smoked (the primary cause).

4. Decreased exercise tolerance—present in Sally Begay
Wheezing
Shortness of breath—present in Sally Begay

5. Pneumonia is an acute infection of the lung caused by bacteria or viruses. Individuals at risk for pneumonia are the young, the very old, or individuals with impaired immunity or underlying disease. Sally Begay has underlying pulmonary disease, which increases her risk. Ira Bradley has impaired immunity, which increases his risk.

6. An unidentified bacterium has caused Sally Begay's pneumonia—probably *Streptococcus pneumoniae*, the most common cause of community acquired pneumonia.
Ira Bradley's pneumonia is caused by *Pneumocystis carinii*, a nonbacterial organism that causes pneumonia in immunocompromised hosts.

7. Pathologic microorganisms enter the lungs by the following routes:
   • When an infected individual coughs, sneezes, or talks, microorganisms are released into the air to be inhaled by others.
   • Microorganisms can be inspired with aerosols (nebulized gas) from contaminated respiratory therapy equipment.
   • In illness or poor dental hygiene, normal flora in the oropharynx can become pathogenic.
   • Staphylococci and gram-negative bacteria can be spread by the circulation from a systemic infection, sepsis, or contaminated needles of intravenous drug abusers.

8.

Signs and Symptoms	Ira Bradley	Sally Begay
Fever	X	X
Chills		
Malaise	X	X
Cough—dry or productive		X
Pleural pain	X	X
Dyspnea	X	X
Hemoptysis		
Elevated white blood cell count		X
Purulent sputum		
Infiltrates on x-ray	X	X

9. The chest x-ray shows fibril calcific involvement of both upper lobes, with pleural thickening bilaterally and blunted costophrenic angles.

10. Yes, because individuals with AIDS are highly susceptible to tuberculosis.

11. Pulmonary embolism

12. Pulmonary embolism

13. A pulmonary embolism is occlusion of a portion of the pulmonary vascular bed by an embolus—a thrombus (blood clot), tissue fragments, or lipids (fats). The impact or effect of the embolus depends on the extent of pulmonary blood flow obstruction, the size of the affected vessels, the nature of the embolus, and the secondary effects. Depending on its pattern of occurrence and severity, pulmonary embolism causes varying degrees of hypoxic vasoconstriction, pulmonary edema, decreased surfactant, atelectasis, and release of neurohormonal substances such as histamine, serotonin, and thromboxane. The embolus also may cause systemic hypotension, decreased cardiac output, and pulmonary hypertension, which, if severe, results in acute right ventricular failure and death.

14. Yes. David Ruskin has right-sided chest pain.

15. Prevent venous stasis through leg elevation, bed exercises, position changes, early postoperative ambulation, and pneumatic calf compression. Clot formation is prevented through anticoagulation.

Lesson 22—Alterations of Renal and Urinary Tract Function

1. Neurogenic bladder

2.

Type	Cause
Uninhibited	Lack of voluntary control in infancy
	Multiple sclerosis
Reflex or automatic	Spinal cord transection
	Cord tumors
	Multiple sclerosis above level T12
Autonomous	Sacral cord trauma
	Tumors
	Herniated disc
	Abdominal surgery with transection of pelvic parasympathetic nerves.
Motor paralysis	Lesions at levels S2, S3, S4
	Poliomyelitis
	Trauma
	Tumors

	Posterior lumbar nerve roots
Sensory paralysis	Diabetes mellitus
	Tabes dorsalis

3. Andrea Wang is at risk for reflex neurogenic bladder.

4. Neurogenic bladder can lead to deterioration of renal function.

5.
Type	**Causes**
Prerenal	Any condition that causes hypovolemia, hypotension, or hypoperfusion
Intrarenal	Acute tubular necrosis
	Glomerulopathies
	Malignant hypertension
	Coagulation defects
Postrenal	Obstructive uropathies

6. Andrea Wang is at risk for postrenal renal failure.

7. Oliguria, elevated BUN and creatinine, electrolyte imbalance, fluid retention (edema), nausea, vomiting, and fatigue

8. No. none of these patients has a UTI.

9. Ira Bradley has a past history of UTI.

10. Both a longer urethra and prostate secretions decrease the risk for UTI in men.

11. Frequency, urgency, dysuria (painful urination), and pain in the suprapubic region or lower back.

12. Carmen Gonzales—because she has diabetes mellitus
Ira Bradley—because he is immunocompromised
Andrea Wang—because she has a neurogenic bladder

13. No. Type 1 (insulin-dependent) diabetes mellitus, not type 2 DM, is a secondary cause of chronic glomerular injury.

Lesson 23—Alterations of Digestive Function

1.
Clinical Manifestations	**Carmen Gonzales**	**Ira Bradley**
Anorexia	X	X
Vomiting	X	
Constipation		
Diarrhea		X
Abdominal pain		
GI bleeding		

2. Overnutrition

3. Ischemic heart disease—Carmen Gonzales has this.
Hyperlipidemia—Carmen Gonzales probably has this, although her lipids were not tested.
Hypertension—Carmen Gonzales has this.
Glucose intolerance—Carmen Gonzales has type 2 diabetes mellitus, so she has this.

4. Decreased calorie intake and increased energy expenditure

5. Starvation

6. Malabsorption syndromes
   Chronic diseases of the cardiovascular, pulmonary, hepatic, and digestive systems—
   Ira Bradley's AIDS affects all of these systems.
   Cancer—Ira Bradley has Kaposi's sarcoma.

7. Enteral or parenteral nutrition

8. Cushing ulcer is a stress ulcer associated with severe head trauma and brain surgery. This ulcer results from decreased mucosal blood flow and hypersecretion of acid caused by overstimulation of the vagal nuclei. Excessive acid damages the mucosal barrier and causes ulceration.

9. Risk factors for gallstones are obesity, middle-age status, female gender, Native American ancestry, and gallbladder, pancreatic, or ileal disease.

10. Sally Begay is at greatest risk for gallstones because she is middle-aged, female, and Native American.

Lesson 24—Alterations of Musculoskeletal Function

1. | Complete | Definition or Distinguishing Characteristics |
|---|---|
| Closed | Noncommunicating wound between bone and skin |
| Open | Communicating wound between bone and skin |
| Comminuted | Multiple bone fragments |
| Linear | Fracture line parallel to long axis of the bone |
| Oblique | Fracture line at 45° angle to long axis of the bone |
| Spiral | Fracture line encircling the bone |
| Transverse | Fracture line perpendicular to long axis of the bone |
| Impacted | Fracture fragments are pushed into one another |
| Pathologic | Fracture occurs at a point in the bone weakened by disease |
| Avulsion | A fragment of bone connected to a ligament or tendon breaks off from the main bone |
| Compression | Fracture is wedged or squeezed together on one side of bone |
| Displaced | Fracture with one, both, or all fragments out of normal alignment |
| Extracapsular | Fragment is close to the joint but remains outside the joint capsule |
| Intracapsular | Fragment is within the joint capsule |

Incomplete	Definition or Distinguishing Characteristics
Greenstick	Break in one cortex of the bone with splintering of inner bone surface
Torus	Buckling of cortex
Bowing	Bending of the bone
Stress	Microfracture
Transchondral	Separation of the cartilaginous joint surface from main shaft of the bone

2. Comminuted fracture of the distal third of the humerus

3. Burst (compression) fracture of T6 and fracture of left posterior lateral sixth rib

4. | Clinical Manifestations | Andrea Wang | David Ruskin |
|---|---|---|
| Impaired function | X | X |
| Unnatural alignment (deformity) | X | X |
| Swelling | X | |
| Muscle spasm | X | |
| Tenderness | X | |
| Pain | X | |
| Impaired sensation | | X |

5. Closed manipulation, traction, and open manipulation

6. Open reduction

7. Open reduction

8. Ligaments, tendons, and muscles

9. Myoglobinuria or rhabdomyolysis

10. Check for dark, reddish-brown urine

11. Contractures, stress-induced muscle tension, fibromyalgia, and disuse atrophy

12. **Contractures**—muscle shortening in the absence of muscle action potential in the sarcolemma
    Disuse atrophy—the pathologic reduction of normal size of muscle fibers after prolonged inactivity

13. Osteomyelitis

14. Bone contains multiple microscopic channels that are impermeable to the cells and biochemicals of the body's natural defenses. Once bacteria gain access to these channels, they are able to proliferate unimpeded.

    The microcirculation of bone is highly vulnerable to damage and destruction by bacterial toxins. Vessel damage causes local thrombosis of the small vessels, which leads to ischemic necrosis of bone.

    Bone cells have a limited capacity to replace bone destroyed by infections. Initially, osteoclasts are stimulated by infection to resorb bone, which opens up isolated bone channels so that cells of the inflammatory and immune system can gain access to the infected bone. At the same time, however, resorption weakens the structural integrity of the bone. New bone formation usually lags behind resorption, and the haversian systems in the new bone are incomplete.

15. Bacteria, fungi, parasites, and viruses

16. **Exogenous**—infection that enters from outside of body through open fractures, penetrating wounds, or surgical procedures
    Endogenous—caused by pathogens carried in the blood from sites of infection elsewhere in the body
    Carmen Gonzales has exogenous osteomyelitis.

17.
Clinical Manifestations	Carmen Gonzales
Fever	X
Malaise	X
Anorexia	X
Weight loss	
Inflammatory exudate	X
Lymphadenopathy	X
Swelling at wound site	X

18.
Treatments	Carmen Gonzales
Antibiotics	X
Drainage of the inflammatory exudate	X
Hyperbaric oxygen	

Lesson 25—Structure, Function, and Disorders of the Integument

1. **Epidermis**—the most important layer of the skin; normally very thin (0.12 mm) but can thicken and form corns and calluses with constant pressure or friction
   Dermis—irregular connective tissue layer with rich blood, lymphatic, and nerve supply; contains sensory receptors and special glands

2. Excoriation

3. Andrea Wang is at risk for pressure ulcers—ischemic ulcers resulting from pressure and shearing forces, which usually develop over bony prominences. Unrelieved pressure causes the endothelial cells lining the capillaries to become disrupted with platelet aggregation, forming microthrombi that block blood flow and cause anoxic necrosis of surrounding tissues. No evidence of pressure ulcers is documented in Andrea Wang's data from 0700 to 1100 on Tuesday.

4. Cellulitis

5. The signs and symptoms are erythema, swelling, and pain. Carmen Gonzales exhibits all of these.

6. Risk factors for candidiasis:
   - A local environment of moisture, warmth, maceration, or occlusion
   - Systemic administration of antibiotics
   - Pregnancy
   - Diabetes mellitus
   - Cushing disease
   - Debilitated states
   - Age younger than 6 months
   - Immunosuppression
   - Certain neoplastic diseases of the blood and monocyte/macrophage system
   - Sexual intercourse with an infected person
   - Inhaled steroids

7. Ira Bradley has an oral candidiasis infection. He is susceptible to such infections because of his immunosuppression and debilitated state.

8. Carmen Gonzales is at risk because of her diabetes mellitus and systemic administration of antibiotics.
   Andrea Wang is at risk because her limited mobility may create local environments of moisture, warmth, maceration, or occlusion.
   Sally Begay is at risk because she is receiving systemic administration of antibiotics.

9. Risk factors for skin cancer:
   - Excessive exposure to ultraviolet radiation from the sun.
   - Fair complexion
   - Occupational exposure to coal tar, pitch, creosote, arsenic compounds, and radium
   - Exposure to human papillomavirus and human immunodeficiency virus

10. Ira Bradley is at risk because he has HIV.
    Sally Begay is at risk because she is a farmer and has excessive exposure to ultraviolet radiation. However she does have protective effects from skin pigmentation (melanin) and from the traditional dress of Native Americans, which protects skin from direct sunlight.

11. Areas widely expose to the sun's rays are the face, head, neck, and hands.

12. Basal cell carcinoma is a surface epithelial tumor of the skin originating from undifferentiated basal or germinative cells. The tumors grow upward and laterally or downward to the dermal epidermal junction. They usually have depressed centers and rolled borders. Early tumors are so small that they are not clinically apparent. Generally, these tumors do not invade blood or lymph vessels; thus they do not metastasize beyond the skin. However basal cell carcinoma can cause severe local destruction. Lesions are seen most frequently in regions of intense sunlight and on those areas most exposed, mainly the face and neck. These tumors arise in consequence to a defect that prevents the cells from being shed by the normal keratinization process. The growth rate of these tumors is quite slow. The lesion starts as a nodule that is pearly or ivory in appearance and slightly elevated above the skin surface with small blood vessels on the surface. As the lesion grows, it often ulcerates, develops crusting, and is firm to the touch. If left untreated, basal cell lesions invade surrounding tissues, and over months or years, can destroy a nose, an eyelid, or and ear.

13. Avoid direct sunlight from 10 a.m. to 3 p.m., when ultraviolet rays are strongest.
    Use sunscreen preparations.
    Examine skin frequently for signs of skin cancer.

14. Ira Bradley has Kaposi's sarcoma, a vascular malignancy. It has several different presentations:
    • In association with drug-induced immunosuppression
    • An endemic form in equatorial Africa
    • A form presenting on the lower legs of elderly men
    • In association with AIDS
    The human immunodeficiency virus and cytomegalovirus have been proposed as cofactors in the development of Kaposi's sarcoma. The herpesvirus may also promote AIDS-related Kaposi's sarcoma. The endothelial cell is thought to be the progenitor of Kaposi's sarcoma. The lesions emerge as purplish brown macules and develop into plaques and nodules. They tend to be multifocal rather than metastatic. The lesions initially appear over the lower extremities in the classic form. The rapidly progressing form associated with AIDS tends to spread symmetrically over the upper body, particularly the face and oral mucosa. The lesions are often pruritic and painful. About 75% of individuals with epidemic Kaposi's sarcoma have involvement of the lymph nodes, particularly in the gastrointestinal tract and lungs. Organ involvement is much less common in the classic form. The rapidly progressive form has a poor prognosis and shorter survival rates than the classic form.
    Ira Bradley seems to have the classic form with a lesion on his leg, although with AIDS, you would more likely expect the rapidly progressing form.

15. Keloids are sharply elevated, irregularly shaped, progressively enlarging scars caused by excessive amounts of collagen in the corneum during connective tissue repair. Ethnic groups particularly at risk are African Americans and Asian Americans. Therefore David Ruskin and Andrea Wang are at risk to develop keloids.

Lesson 26—Shock, Multiple Organ Dysfunction Syndrome, and Burns in Adults

1. Cardiogenic shock results from heart failure of any cause. Most cases of cardiogenic shock follow myocardial infarction or surgery requiring cardiopulmonary bypass. Shock also can follow heart failure from any cause, myocardial stunning, myocardial ischemia, myocardial or pericardial infections, dysrhythmias, tension pneumothorax, and conditions causing excessive right ventricular afterload. Cardiogenic shock is notoriously unresponsive to treatment, with inhospital mortalities of 71% reported. As cardiac output decreases, renal and hypothalamic adaptive responses maintain or increase blood volume. Blood pressure is maintained through vasoconstriction in response to catecholamine release from the adrenals. Catecholamines also increase contractility and heart rate. Increases in blood‚volume and vascular resistance succeed in normalizing blood pressure and increasing cardiac performance—but at the cost of increasing myocardial demands for oxygen and nutrients. Increas-

ing myocardial requirements further strain the already failing heart, which can no longer pump an adequate volume of blood with sufficient force to perfuse the tissues. The direct effect of decreased tissue perfusion is impaired cellular metabolism.

2. Patients at risk for cardiogenic shock:
Sally Begay, who has congestive heart failure and a history of myocardial infarction
Carmen Gonzales, who has congestive heart failure

3. Impaired mentation, elevated preload in the systemic and pulmonary vasculature, systemic and pulmonary edema, low cardiac output, dusky skin color, low blood pressure, oliguria, ileus, and dyspnea

4. Andrea Wang has neurogenic shock, a widespread and massive vasodilation that results from an imbalance between parasympathetic and sympathetic stimulation of vascular smooth muscle. Occasionally parasympathetic overstimulation or sympathetic understimulation persists, causing vasodilation for an extended period. Extreme, persistent vasodilation leads to neurogenic shock. Neurogenic shock creates "relative hypovolemia." Blood volume has not changed, but the amount of space containing the blood has increased, so SVR decreases drastically. With a decreased SVR, pressure in the vessels is inadequate to drive nutrients across capillary membranes and nutrient delivery to the cells is impaired. As with other types of shock, this leads to impaired cellular metabolism. Neurogenic shock can be caused by any factor that stimulates parasympathetic activity or inhibits sympathetic activity of vascular smooth muscle. Normally, sympathetic stimulation maintains muscle tone. If sympathetic stimulation is interrupted or inhibited, vasodilation occurs. Therefore trauma to the spinal cord or medulla, conditions that interrupt the supply of oxygen to the medulla, or conditions that deprive the medulla of glucose all cause neurogenic shock by interrupting sympathetic activity.

5. The clinical manifestations of neurogenic shock are bradycardia and hypotension. Andrea Wang exhibits both of these.

6. Stabilization of the spine and surrounding tissues is the beginning treatment. Andrea Wang was taken directly from the emergency department to the operating room for spinal stabilization.

7. Septic shock begins with a nidus of infection that may be readily discernible or extremely difficult to locate. Bacteria then enter the bloodstream to produce bacteremia in one of two ways:
 • Directly from the site of infection
 • From toxic substances released by bacteria directly into the bloodstream
   These toxic substances, which act as triggering molecules in the septic syndrome, include endotoxins produced by gram-negative microorganisms, teichoic acid antigen produced by gram-positive microorganisms, and exotoxins. The triggering molecules cause the host to initiate a nonspecific, first-line defense response using phagocytic cells and the complement cascade. Shortly after this response, a specific immune response is initiated with the release of primary mediators. Release of these mediators triggers intense cellular responses and subsequent release of secondary mediators. Chemotaxis, activation of the granulocytes, and reactivation of phagocytic cells and the inflammatory cascade result. The patient frequently progresses from septic shock to multiple organ dysfunction syndrome (MODS) following the release of secondary mediators.

8. The patients at risk for septic shock are those with infections—Ira Bradley, Sally Begay, and Carmen Gonzales.

9. Risk factors for MODS:
 • Age over 65 years
 • Baseline organ dysfunction

- Bowel infarction
- Coma on admission
- Inadequate or delayed resuscitation
- Malnutrition
- Multiple blood transfusions
- Persistent infectious focus
- Preexisting chronic disease
- Presence of hematoma
- Significant tissue injury
- Use of steroids

10. Ira Bradley is at highest risk for MODS, because he has baseline organ dysfunction, malnutrition, persistent infectious focus, and preexisting chronic disease.
    Carmen Gonzales is also at risk for MODS, because she has a persistent infectious focus and preexisting chronic disease.

onRamp
to
Algebra.™

Extra Practice Workbook

PEARSON

Boston, Massachusetts • Chandler, Arizona • Glenview, Illinois • Upper Saddle River, New Jersey

ISBN-13:   978-0-13-322862-5
ISBN-10:   0-13-322862-2
11 19

Table of Contents

Table of Contents

UNIT 4 Ratio and Proportionality

Table of Contents

1-1   Reasoning with Diagrams

Extra Practice

1. Each of these diagrams represents a numerical expression using multiplication. Write the numerical expression using numbers and a symbol for multiplication.

a.

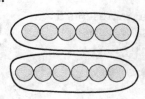

_____

b.

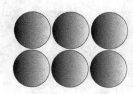

_____

c.

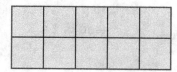

_____

d.

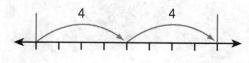

_____

e.

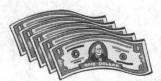

_____

2. a. Sketch a diagram, like the one in Problem 1(a), that represents 6×2 instead of 2×6.

Extra Practice continued _____

    b. How do the diagrams in 1(a) and 2(a) show different expressions for the same value?

_____

_____

_____

    c. Write an equation showing that the amounts in the diagrams are equal.

_____

3. a. Sketch a diagram, like the one in Problem 1(c), that represents 5×2 instead of 2×5.

    b. How do the diagrams in 1(c) and 3(a) show different expressions for the same value?

_____

_____

_____

    c. Write an equation showing that the amounts in the diagrams are equal.

_____

Reasoning with Numbers

Extra Practice

Problems 1–3 contain statements classified as *always true*, *sometimes true*, or *never true*. Each statement is followed by a justification.

Decide whether each justification is convincing. Rewrite the justifications that are not convincing. Use a diagram, definitions, and/or properties of numbers in your justification.

1. When you subtract one number from another number, the result is an odd number.

    This statement is *sometimes true*.

    Justification: $12 - 10 = 2$.   The number 2 is even, not odd.

    $\qquad\qquad\quad 12 - 11 = 1$.   The number 1 is odd.

    a. If this justification is convincing, explain. If the justification is not convincing, rewrite it.

    _____

    _____

    b. Can you explain when the statement is true? What types of numbers make this true?

    _____

    _____

    _____

Extra Practice continued

2. When you multiply any odd number by 2, the result is an odd number.

   This statement is *never true*.

   Justification: When you multiply any number of items by 2, the result can be arranged so that each item is paired with another.

   $$2 \times \bigcirc\bigcirc\bigcirc\bigcirc\bigcirc = \begin{matrix}\circ\circ\circ\circ\circ\\\circ\circ\circ\circ\circ\end{matrix} \quad \text{or} \quad$$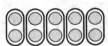

   There will be no unpaired item, or remainder. A number that can be divided into pairs with no remainder is even. *Even* is defined as a whole number that is divisible by 2. And a number property states: no number is both even and odd.

   If this justification is convincing, explain. Otherwise, rewrite it.

   _____

   _____

3. When you multiply any even number by 2, the result is an even number.

   This statement is *always true*.

   Justification: $6 \times 2 = 12$, $8 \times 2 = 16$, $10 \times 2 = 20$, and so on.

   If this justification is convincing, explain. Otherwise, rewrite it.

   _____

   _____

   _____

4. The following statement is *sometimes true*.

   When you add more than two odd numbers, the sum is odd.

   Make a diagram that illustrates that the statement can be *false*.

   Possible solution

1-3 Reasoning with Variables

Extra Practice

A table is a good way to organize data. When you have more than one value, you can use a table to show which values go together.

1. This table shows some values for *a* and 3*a*.

a	4	5	6	12	15	120
3*a*	12	15	18	36	45	360

a. Make a table like the one above that shows other values for *a* and 3*a*.

b. Does your table include all of the possible values for *a* and 3*a*? If it does, say how you know. If it does not, explain whether it is possible to make a table that includes all the possible values for *a* and 3*a*.

_____

_____

2. If any number *a* is multiplied by 3, and then 3 is added to the result, the amount can be written as the algebraic expression 3*a* + 3. Calculate the value of 3*a* + 3 for each value of *a*.

a. *a* = 1   **b.** *a* = 2   **c.** *a* = 3

_____   _____   _____

Extra Practice continued

3. Make a table showing values for *a* and 3*a* + 3. Choose any five values for *a* and then calculate the value of 3*a* + 3 for each value of *a*.

4. Think about this statement: If *a* is an odd number, then 3*a* is an odd number.

Is this statement *always true*, *sometimes true*, or *never true*? Justify your choice mathematically.

_____

_____

_____

_____

_____

5. Think about this statement: If *a* is an odd number, then 3*a* + 3 is an odd number.

Is this statement *always true*, *sometimes true*, or *never true*? Justify your choice mathematically.

_____

_____

_____

_____

1-4 Conventions for Using Numbers and Variables

Extra Practice

1. a. Express "nine multiplied by *x*" using conventions.   _____

   b. If *x* = 6, what does 9*x* equal?   _____

   c. Write "*a* multiplied by twenty-four" as an algebraic expression.   _____

   d. If *a* = 3, what does 24*a* equal?   _____

Sample

What does 8*n* mean? 8*n* means "eight multiplied by *n*."

Suppose *n* is 5, then 8*n* is 8 · 5, or 40.

So, if *n* = 5, then 8*n* = 40.

2. a. Write "*a* multiplied by *b*" as an algebraic expression.   _____

   b. If *a* = 16 and *b* = 3, what does *a* multiplied by *b* equal?   _____

Sample

What does *xy* mean? *xy* means *x* multiplied by *y*.

Suppose *x* is 2 and *y* is 3, then *xy* is 2 · 3, or 6.

So, if *x* = 2 and *y* = 3, then *xy* = 6.

Extra Practice continued _____

3. a. Express "twenty-four divided by *a*" using conventions. _____

  b. If *a* = 6, what does "24 divided by *a*" equal? _____

  c. Write "*b* divided by *a*" as an algebraic expression. _____

Sample

What does $\frac{8}{n}$ mean? $\frac{8}{n}$ means 8 divided by *n*.

Suppose *n* is 4, then $\frac{8}{n}$ is $8 \div 4$, or 2.

So, if $n = 4$, then $\frac{8}{n} = 2$.

4. a. Write "*a* divided by twenty-four" as an algebraic expression. _____

  b. If *a* = 6, what does "*a* divided by 24" equal? _____

  c. Write "*a* divided by *b*" as an algebraic expression. _____

5. Let *m* = 18 and *n* = 9.

  a. Calculate the value of "*m* divided by *n*." _____

  b. Calculate the value of "*n* divided by *m*." _____

1-5 Conventions for Using Parentheses

Extra Practice

1. Calculate the value of each numerical expression.

   a. $(3 \cdot 6) \div (6 - 3)$

   _____

   b. $5(3 + 2) \div (2 \cdot 5)$

   _____

2. **a.** Use parentheses and the $\cdot$ and $\div$ symbols to rewrite $\dfrac{5 \times 9}{3 \times 6}$. _____

   b. Calculate the value of the numerical expression. _____

   c. Why is it appropriate to use the $\cdot$ symbol in this problem, but not in $\dfrac{5n}{3m}$?

   _____

   _____

   _____

3. Write an algebraic expression for each statement. If necessary, use parentheses to make the meaning of the expression clear.

   a. An unknown number is multiplied by 5, and 3 is added to the result. _____

   b. The number 3 is added to an unknown number, and the result is multiplied by 5. _____

Extra Practice continued

4. a. Using parentheses and a fraction bar, rewrite the algebraic expression $a \div b - 2$ in two ways that each give a different result.

_____

b. Substitute the values $a = 10$ and $b = 5$ into each algebraic expression. Calculate the value of each expression.

_____

_____

5. A student using a calculator multiplied a number n by 4 and then divided the result by 10. The number 400 appeared in the calculator display.

Suppose the student had first divided the number n by 10 and then multiplied the result by 4. What number would appear in the calculator display? Say how you know.

_____

_____

_____

6. Rosa said that the perimeter of this rectangle can be represented by the algebraic expression $2h + 14$.

Jamal said the perimeter is $2(h + 7)$.

Who is correct? Justify your answer.

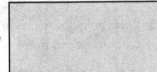

h

7

_____

_____

_____

The Number Properties

🟦 Extra Practice

1. Write an equation with numbers (no variables) that shows each property.

   a. Commutative Property of Multiplication   _____

   b. Associative Property of Addition   _____

   c. Identity Property of Addition   _____

   d. Commutative Property of Addition   _____

   e. Associative Property of Multiplication   _____

   f. Identity Property of Multiplication   _____

🟦 Sample

Commutative Property of Multiplication $2 \cdot 3 = 3 \cdot 2$

2. Dwayne said that the equation $10 \div 20 = 20 \div 10$ is true because $10 \div 20$ has the same value as $20 \div 10$. Rosa said that the equation is false because $10 \div 20$ does not have the same value as $20 \div 10$.

   Who is correct? Say why.

   _____

   _____

Extra Practice continued

3. Say whether each equation is true or false. For each false equation, explain why it is false.

a. $\frac{15}{3+2} = 15 \div (3+2)$

_____

_____

b. $\frac{15}{3+2} = 15 \div 3 + 2$

_____

_____

c. $\frac{15}{3} + 2 = 15 \div 3 + 2$

_____

_____

d. $\frac{15}{3} + 2 = 15 \div (3+2)$

_____

_____

_____

1-7 Conventions and the Number Properties

Extra Practice

1. Say whether each equation is true or false. For each equation that is true, write the number property shown by the equation.

   a. $7 \cdot 1 = 7$

   _____

   b. $(5 + 9) + 1 = 5 + (9 + 1)$

   _____

   _____

   c. $9 - 4 = 4 - 9$

   _____

   d. $6 + 0 = 6$

   _____

   e. $(4 \cdot 2) \cdot 6 = 4 \cdot (2 \cdot 6)$

   _____

   _____

   f. $10 \div 1 = 1 \div 10$

   _____

Extra Practice continued

2. Let $x = 4$. What is the value of y if:

   a. $y = 2x$ **b.** $y = 4x$ **c.** $y = 5x$

   _____   _____   _____

3. An equilateral triangle is a triangle with three sides of equal length. The perimeter of an equilateral triangle is defined as *Perimeter* = 3 • *side length*. You can write this with variables as $P = 3s$.

Suppose the perimeter of an equilateral triangle is 24 inches.

You can write this as $24 = 3s$.

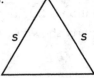

Given	Need
$P = 24$ in.	$s = ?$

What is the value of s? Explain how you know.

_____

_____

4. This table gives the perimeter of several different equilateral triangles.

   a. Fill in the side length for each equilateral triangle.

Perimeter (in.)	6	9	18	30	45	n
Number of Sides	3	3	3	3	3	3
Side Length (in.)						

   b. What is the rule for finding the side length of an equilateral triangle when the perimeter is known? Give the rule in words and write an equation.

_____

_____

1-8 Using Variables in Formulas

Extra Practice

1. Calculate the height of a rectangle with area $A = 28$ square units for each base b.

   a. $b = 4$ units   **b.** $b = 14$ units   **c.** $b = x$ units

   _____   _____   _____

2. The rule for calculating the area of a rectangle is *Area = base • height*. You can write this rule using the formula $A = bh$. Explain in words how to calculate the length of the base if you are given the area and height of a rectangle.

   _____

   _____

3. **a.** Each of these rectangles has an area of 24 square units. Make a table showing the height, base, and area of these four rectangles.

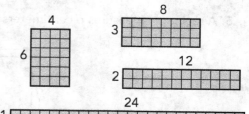

   b. Write a general formula to calculate the base b of a rectangle if you know the height h and that the area is 24 (square units).

   _____

Extra Practice continued

4. The perimeter of a figure is the distance around its outer edge.

  a. Write a description of how you would calculate the perimeter of a rectangle when $b = 4$ cm and $h = 2$ cm.

  _____

  _____

  b. Calculate the perimeter of a rectangle when $b = 12$ cm and $h = 6$ cm.   _____

  c. Write a formula for the perimeter of a rectangle. Let b stand for base and h for height.

  _____

Sample

For a rectangle with a base of 3 units and a height of 2 units, the perimeter is $3 + 3 + 2 + 2 = 10$ units.

For a rectangle with a base of 6 units and a height of 4 units, the perimeter is $6 + 6 + 4 + 4 = 20$ units.

5. A rectangle measures d centimeters by 6 centimeters.

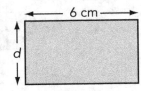

  a. Write a formula to represent the area of the rectangle.   _____

  b. Write a formula to represent the perimeter of the rectangle.   _____

1-9 The Distributive Property

■ Extra Practice

1. Substitute each set of numbers in the equation $a(b + c) = ab + ac$, and calculate the value of each side separately to be sure that the equation is true.

   a. $a = 5, b = 9, c = 4$

   _____

   _____

   _____

   b. $a = 5, b = 6, c = 8$

   _____

   _____

   _____

   c. $a = 8, b = 5, c = 6$

   _____

   _____

2. Sketch number lines that represent both sides of the equation $3(1 + 4) = (3 \cdot 1) + (3 \cdot 4)$.

3. Use the Distributive Property to rewrite these expressions.

   a. $3(9 - 5)$

   _____

   _____

   b. $2(x + 8)$

   _____

   _____

Extra Practice continued

4. Sketch a diagram of each rectangle. Show the Distributive Property by
   calculating the area of each rectangle in two different ways.

   a. height = 5

   base = 3 + 4

   b. height = 4

   base = $x + 2$

   _____   _____

   _____   _____

   _____   _____

5. Use the Distributive Property to rewrite each expression as the product of a
   number or variable and a quantity in parentheses.

   a. $5a + 5b$ **b.** $(4 \cdot 2) + (4 \cdot 7)$ **c.** $3x + 4x$

   _____   _____   _____

Sample

Start with the expression $2a + 2b$. The number 2 is multiplied by both a and b.
Using the Distributive Property, you can write $2a + 2b$ as $2(a + b)$.

6. The expression $9 \cdot 27$ can be written as $9 \cdot (25 + 2)$. How else could you
   write this expression? Which expression do you find easiest to solve?
   Explain.

   _____

   _____

   _____

1-10 Applying the Distributive Property

📋 Extra Practice

1. **a.** A student wrote: $a(b + c) = ab + c$. What mistake did the student make?

   _____

   _____

   b. Sketch an area model and use it to describe why the equation is not true.

   _____

   _____

2. List the number properties that justify each step. Four steps can be justified by simple arithmetic. In these cases, name the operation that justifies the step.

   Justification

   $19 \cdot 23 = 19(20 + 3)$ _____

   $\qquad = (19 \cdot 20) + (19 \cdot 3)$ _____

   $\qquad = (20 \cdot 19) + (3 \cdot 19)$ _____

   $\qquad = 20(10 + 9) + 3(10 + 9)$ _____

   $\qquad = (20 \cdot 10) + (20 \cdot 9) + (3 \cdot 10)$ _____
   $\qquad \quad + (3 \cdot 9)$
   $\qquad = 200 + 180 + 30 + 27$ _____

   $\qquad = 437$ _____

Extra Practice continued

3. Suppose you cannot remember the product of 8 and 9. How can you use expanded form and the Distributive Property to help you multiply 8 • 9?

_____

4. Use expanded form and the Distributive Property to multiply 39 • 64.

_____

_____

5. In the expression $9a + 9b$, 9 is multiplied by both a and b. Using parentheses, you can write $9a + 9b$ as $9(a + b)$. Rewrite each expression in the same way.

   a. $2x + 2y$ **b.** $6x + 6$ **c.** $5y + 9y$ **d.** $ab + bc$

   _____   _____   _____   _____

6. Sketch an area model to support your multiplication of 39 • 64 in Problem 4.

7. Multiply $(x + 6)(y + 7)$. Sketch an area model that represents this calculation.

_____

_____

The Inverses of Addition and Multiplication

Extra Practice

1. What is the inverse of each of these operations?

   a. Dividing by 12

   _____

   b. Multiplying by $\frac{1}{5}$

   _____

   c. Adding $\frac{3}{4}$

   _____

2. $-a$ is the additive inverse of a.

   $\frac{1}{a}$ is the multiplicative inverse of a.

   a. What is the additive inverse of 5? _____

   b. What is the additive inverse of -5? _____

   c. What is the multiplicative inverse of 5? _____

   d. What is the multiplicative inverse of $\frac{1}{5}$? _____

Extra Practice continued

3. Write the value of *a* that makes each of these equations true.

a. $\frac{1}{5}a = 1$

b. $\frac{1}{5}a = 5$

c. $\frac{1}{5}a = 10$

_____

_____

_____

d. $\frac{1}{5}a = 20$

e. $\frac{1}{5}a = 100$

f. $5a = 100$

_____

_____

_____

4. Write a description of how to calculate the values of *a* in Problem 3 using inverses.

_____

_____

_____

_____

_____

_____

1-12 Progress Check

Extra Practice

1. Correct the equations that are not true and give the number property that each corrected equation represents. Note: There is more than one way to correct each equation. Try not to use the same property twice.

a. $9 + 0 = 0$

_____

b. $9 - 9 = 9$

_____

c. $9 \cdot \frac{1}{9} = 9$

_____

d. $9 \cdot 1 = 1$

_____

e. $9 + 3 = 3 - 9$

_____

f. $9 \cdot 3 = 3 \div 9$

_____

g. $9 + (3 + 10) = (9 + 3) + (9 + 10)$

_____

h. $9(3 \cdot 10) = (9 \cdot 3) + (9 \cdot 10)$

_____

Extra Practice continued

2. Substitute each set of values for *a*, *b*, and *c* in the equation $a(b + c) = ab + ac$. Calculate the value of each side to show that each equation is true.

   a. $a = 10$, $b = \frac{1}{2}$, $c = 1$

   b. $a = 2$, $b = x$, $c = 6$

   _____   _____

   _____   _____

   _____   _____

3. Sketch an area model that represents the Distributive Property for each equation in Problem 2. Label the base and the height of each rectangle.

4. This rectangle has an area of 36 cm². The product of the base *b* and the height *h* is 36 square centimeters. In other words, $bh = 36$ cm².

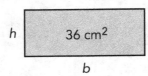

h 36 cm²

b

Complete the table by filling in four possible pairs of values for the base *b* and the height *h* of this rectangle. Remember that the area is 36 cm².

b (cm)	1				
h (cm)	36				

5. Write a formula for the base of the rectangle in Problem 4 in terms of *h*. _____

6. Write a formula for the height of the rectangle in Problem 4 in terms of *b*. _____

1-13 Relationships between Quantities

Extra Practice

1. a. Every dog has four legs. What are the two quantities in this situation?

Number of Dogs	1	2	3	4	5
Number of Legs	4	8	12	16	20

_____

b. Do the quantities vary in relation to each other? In other words, as one quantity increases or decreases, does the other quantity increase or decrease?

_____

c. State another quantity of dogs and calculate the total number of legs.

_____

_____

d. Which statement describes the relationship between the two quantities?

  Ⓐ   The number of dogs is equal to twice the number of legs.

  Ⓑ   The number of dogs is equal to four times the number of legs.

  Ⓒ   The number of legs is equal to four times the number of dogs.

  Ⓓ   The number of legs is equal to the number of dogs plus three.

e. Which formula (where d stands for the number of dogs and l stands for the number of legs) gives the number of legs in terms of the number of dogs?

  Ⓐ $d = l$ Ⓑ $d = 2l$ Ⓒ $d = 4l$ Ⓓ $l = 4d$ Ⓔ $l = d + 3$

Extra Practice continued

2. School pictures are ordered in sheets with 8 pictures on 1 sheet.

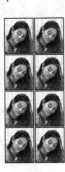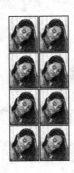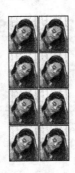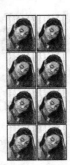

a. How many sheets are shown in the diagram above? _____

b. How many pictures are shown in the diagram above? _____

c. Make a table showing four pairs of values for the number of sheets and the number of pictures.

d. Write a formula for the number of sheets in terms of the number of pictures.

_____

3. A web site is having a special sale. During the sale, all used paperback books cost $1 each. No matter how many books are ordered, the total cost of the order includes a handling fee of $5 and a shipping fee of $4.

a. What two quantities vary in this situation?

_____

_____

b. What is the total cost if you order 5 books? _____

c. How many books did you order if the total cost is $17? _____

d. Write a formula for the total cost in terms of the number of books. _____

1-14 Using Graphs to Represent Relationships

 ## Extra Practice

The figures show a single cup and stack of three cups. The lip of each cup is 1 cm tall, and the rest of the cup is 5 cm tall.

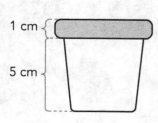

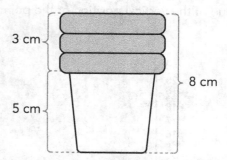

1. The two quantities that vary in relation to each other in this situation are:

   • The number of cups in the stack

   • The height of the stack of cups

   a. What is the height of a stack of 2 of these cups? _____

   b. What is the height of a stack of 5 of these cups? _____

   c. What is the height of a stack of 10 of these cups? _____

2. Make a table showing five pairs of values for the two quantities that vary in this situation. You may include the values you found in Problem 1 or find all new values to include in your table.

Extra Practice continued

3. Represent each pair of values shown in your table as ordered pairs, (*x*, *y*).

- Let *x* stand for the numbers of cups in a stack.

- Let *y* stand for the height of a stack.

_____

4. Label the *x*- and *y*-axes of the graph with the appropriate quantity. Plot and label the points from your table on the graph.

Remember that *x* is the value of the horizontal position of the point, and *y* is the value of the vertical position of the point.

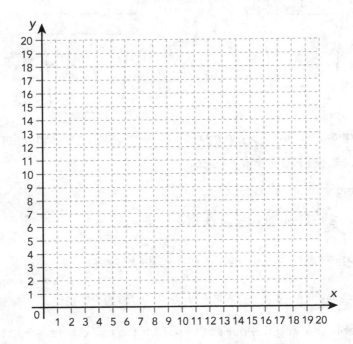

1-15 Understanding the Problem Situation

Extra Practice

Dwayne needs to buy a phone. There are two plans he is thinking about:

PLAN A

$25.00 a month plus 10 cents a minute

Two-year minimum contract

PLAN B

$30.00 a month plus 5 cents a minute

One-year minimum contract

1. Dwayne made some notes about the quantities in Plan A. He wrote:

   1. The charge per month for Plan A is $25.00.

   2. The charge per minute is 10 cents, so multiply the number of minutes by $0.10.

   3. The cost for a month depends on the number of minutes.

      a. Why does Dwayne's second note make sense?

      _____

      _____

      b. Does Dwayne's last note make sense to you? If not, say why not.

      _____

2. Make notes about the quantities in the description of Plan B. Use Dwayne's notes as a model.

   _____

   _____

   _____

   _____

Extra Practice continued _____

3. Dwayne made this table for Plan A.

Number of Minutes	1	10	100	300	400	500
Total Cost per Month	$25.10	$26.00	$35.00	$55.00	$65.00	$75.00

Sketch a graph of this relationship on the coordinate plane. Label the line *Plan A*.

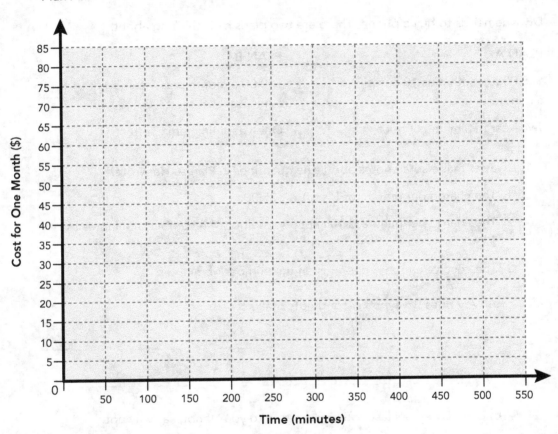

4. Dwayne began this table for Plan B.

Number of Minutes	1	10	100	300	400	500
Total Cost per Month	$30.05	$30.50				

a. Complete the table then sketch a graph of this relationship on the coordinate plane in Problem 3. Label the line *Plan B*.

b. What conclusions can Dwayne make from the graph?

_____

_____

1-16 Representing Problem Situations

Extra Practice

For Problems 1–5, use the following situation.

Carlos volunteers at the local animal shelter. When animals are brought to the shelter, they must be weighed, but it is hard to get the animals to stand still on the scale. To solve this problem, Carlos weighs each animal in his arms. Carlos weighs 173 pounds.

1. In this situation, two quantities vary in relation to each other:

- Weight of each animal, in pounds

- Total weight shown on the scale, in pounds

    a. Assign variables to these quantities.

    _____

    _____

    b. There is another quantity in this situation that does not vary. What is it?

    _____

2. Make a table showing at least four values for each of the quantities that vary in this situation. Use the variables you assigned in Problem 1 to label the rows in your table, and be sure to clearly show which values correspond to each other. Your values should reflect realistic weights for cats and dogs.

Extra Practice continued

3. Which graph best represents the relationship between the quantities?

Ⓐ
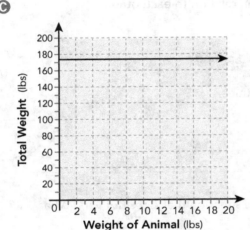

Ⓑ
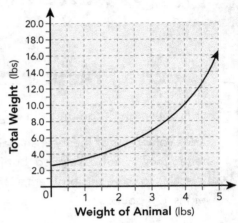

Ⓒ

Ⓓ
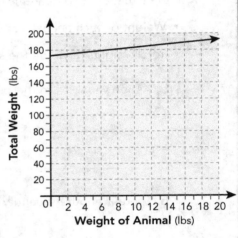

4. Look at the graph you chose in Problem 3. Every point on the graph represents the weight of an animal and the corresponding total weight shown on the scale. For example, the point with coordinates (3, 176) represents a kitten that weighs 3 pounds and the corresponding weight of Carlos plus the kitten.

Find the point (3, 176) on the graph you chose in Problem 3. Then write at least four other points on this graph as ordered pairs. Choose at least one point that has a weight that is not a whole number.

_____

5. Write a formula that represents the relationship between the weight of each animal *W* and the total weight shown on the scale *T*.

_____

1-17 Writing Formulas to Answer Questions

▣ Extra Practice

On Saturday, Rosa, Jamal, Dwayne, Lisa, and Lisa's sister, Annie, decide to go to the park where they can rent bicycles. On weekends, there is a $5 initial fee, plus a rental price of $5 per hour.

Bike Rental
$5 + $5 per hour

1. What are the quantities in this situation? Assign a variable to each one.

_____

_____

_____

_____

2. In this situation, the two quantities that vary in relation to each other are:

- The number of hours a bike is rented
- The price per person to rent the bike

   a. What is the price per person to rent a bike for 1 hour? _____

   b. What is the price per person to rent a bike for 2 hours? _____

   c. What is the price per person to rent a bike for 6 hours? _____

   d. Jamal paid $40 to rent a bike. For how many hours did he rent the bike? _____

   e. Rosa paid $50 to rent a bike. For how many hours did she rent the bike? _____

Extra Practice continued

3. This table shows values of the two quantities that vary in this situation.

Hours Rented	3	4	5	10
Price per Person ($)	20	25	30	55

Give three more pairs of values that could be included in this table.

_____

4. Sketch a graph to represent the relationship between the hours rented and the price per person. Graph three points defined in the table for Problem 3.

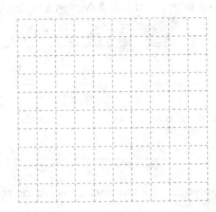

5. Write a formula that tells you how much it costs to rent a bike for *h* hours. _____

6. Use this formula to calculate the total cost when $h = 8$. _____

7. Use this formula to calculate the hours rented if the total cost was $65. _____

8. How would you change this formula if you wanted to know the total cost for all five people to rent bikes for *h* hours? Use the Distributive Property to write a new formula.

_____

1-18 The Unit in Review

Extra Practice

1. **a.** Which value is equal to the expression $3(4 + 8)$?

    (A) 15   (B) 20   (C) 28   (D) 36   (E) 96

    b. Which number property allows you to write $3(4 + 8) = (3 \cdot 4) + (3 \cdot 8)$?

    _____

    c. Sketch an area model to show that $3(4 + 8) = (3 \cdot 4) + (3 \cdot 8)$.

2. Write the expression $\frac{a + 2}{3}$ in words. Use the word "quantity" if it makes your answer clearer. Then find the value of the expression when $a = 7$.

    _____

    _____

3. Name the number property or convention that justifies each statement.

    a. $a + (b + c) = (a + b) + c$

    _____

    b. $a \cdot 1 = a$

    _____

    c. $ab = ba$

    _____

Extra Practice continued

4. Keesha is making apple pies for a school bake sale. Apples cost $1.50 per pound. She makes a table to show the relationship between the weight of apples a in pounds and the cost c in dollars.

   a. Complete the table.

a	1	2	4	5	8
c	$1.50	$3.00			

   b. Write three more pairs of values that could be included in the table. Write the values as ordered pairs.

   _____

   c. Sketch a graph to represent the relationship between the weight of apples and the cost.

   d. Write a formula representing the relationship between the two quantities. _____

   e. How much will it cost to buy n pounds of apples?

   Ⓐ $1 + n$ Ⓑ $n + \$1.50$ Ⓒ $\$1.50n$ Ⓓ $\$1.50$ Ⓔ $15n$

2-1 Adding and Subtracting Fractions

Extra Practice

1. Use addition to write the equation that is represented by each number line. Write the sum in simplest form.

a.

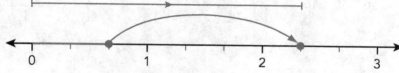

_____

b.

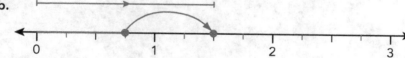

_____

2. Use subtraction to write the equation that is represented by each number line. Write the difference in simplest form.

a.

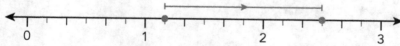

_____

b.

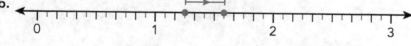

_____

Extra Practice continued _____

3. Use the given number line to sketch a diagram for each calculation. Then write the sum or difference in simplest form.

a. $\frac{4}{5} + \frac{4}{5}$ _____

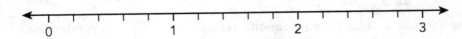

b. $\frac{3}{10} + \frac{3}{10} + \frac{3}{10} + \frac{3}{10} + \frac{3}{10}$ _____

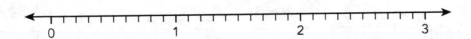

c. $\frac{11}{10} + \frac{9}{10}$ _____

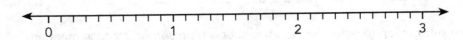

d. $\frac{9}{10} - \frac{7}{10}$ _____

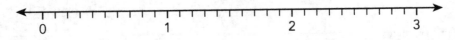

e. $2 - \frac{7}{5}$ _____

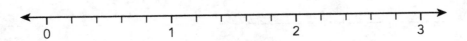

f. $\frac{12}{5} - \frac{6}{5}$ _____

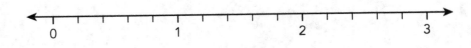

2-2 Adding with Different Denominators

◼ Extra Practice

1. a. Use this number line with a scale marked in twenty-fourths to represent the equation $\frac{15}{24} + \frac{18}{24} = \frac{33}{24}$.

b. Explain why the equation in part (a) is equivalent to $\frac{5}{8} + \frac{3}{4} = \frac{11}{8}$.

_____

2. a. Use this number line with a scale marked in eighteenths to represent the equation $\frac{6}{18} + \frac{8}{18} = \frac{14}{18}$.

b. Write an equivalent equation using smaller denominators.

_____

c. Explain how to make a number line that represents this new equation.

_____

_____

_____

Extra Practice continued

3. a. Use this number line with a scale marked in sixteenths to represent the equation $\frac{8}{16} + \frac{12}{16} = \frac{20}{16}$.

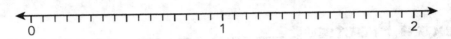

b. Write an equivalent equation using smaller denominators.

_____

c. Explain how to make a number line that represents this new equation.

_____

_____

_____

4. Calculate the value of these expressions, using equivalent fractions. Write your answers in simplest form.

a. $\frac{5}{7} + \frac{3}{4}$

_____

b. $2\frac{5}{7} + \frac{3}{4}$

_____

c. $\frac{5}{8} + \frac{3}{5}$

_____

d. $2\frac{5}{8} + 1\frac{3}{5}$

_____

e. $\frac{5}{20} + \frac{36}{100}$

_____

f. $1\frac{5}{20} + 10\frac{36}{100}$

_____

2-3 Multiplying by a Whole Number

Extra Practice

1. Lisa's class is making a film. In the film, Lisa, whose real height is 5 feet 4 inches, must look like she is 4 feet tall. The students achieve this by building a set in which everything is much bigger than normal.

Lisa's actual height is $\frac{4}{3}$ larger than the size she needs to appear.

$$\frac{5'4''}{4'0''} = \frac{64''}{48''} = \frac{4}{3}$$

For Lisa to appear small, each of the props needs to be scaled to $\frac{4}{3}$ of its actual size.

Complete the table.

Normal Size	Large Set Design Size
Doorway, 90 inches high	
Chair, 36 inches high	
Cup, 9 cm wide	
Plate, 27 cm wide	
Spear, 5 feet 6 inches long	

2. Measure the normal size of three other objects, and then calculate the sizes they would have to be in the large set design. Complete the table.

Normal Size	Large Set Design Size

Extra Practice continued

3. An identical but smaller set must be built for Jamal, whose real height is 5 feet 10 inches. The set design must make Jamal look like he is a 7-foot giant.

   a. Calculate the fraction by which the props must be scaled. (*Hint*: Use Problem 1 as a guide.)

   _____

   _____

   b. Complete the table.

Normal Size	Small Set Design Size
Doorway, 90 inches high	
Chair, 36 inches high	
Cup, 9 cm wide	
Plate, 27 cm wide	
Spear, 5 feet 6 inches long	

4. Represent the following calculations as repeated steps on a number line.

   a. $3 \cdot \frac{3}{5}$

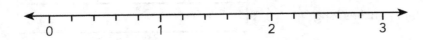

   b. $4 \cdot \frac{2}{3}$

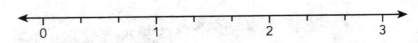

   c. $4 \cdot \frac{7}{15}$

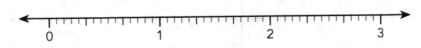

2-4 Multiplying Fractions

▣ Extra Practice

1. Each of these diagrams represents the multiplication of two fractions.

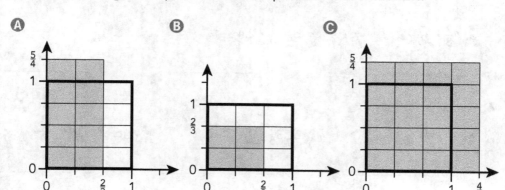

A   **B**   **C**

a. Which area diagram represents $\frac{5}{4} \cdot \frac{4}{3} = \frac{20}{12} = \frac{5}{3}$? _____

b. Write the equation represented by each of the other diagrams.

   • Find the fractions being multiplied on the horizontal and vertical axes.

   • Count the number of rectangles in the unit square and write that as the denominator.

   • Count the number of rectangles in the shaded area and write that as the numerator.

   _____

c. Which diagrams represent fractions less than 1? Explain how this is shown.

   _____

   _____

   _____

   _____

Extra Practice continued

2. Write the following numbers in the form $\frac{a}{b}$, where a and b are whole numbers.

    a. $1\frac{7}{8}$ **b.** $3\frac{1}{5}$ **c.** 2.4

    _____   _____   _____

3. Calculate the value of the following expressions, using the answers to the previous problem and equivalent fractions. Write your answers in simplest form.

    a. $1\frac{7}{8} \cdot 3\frac{1}{5}$ **b.** $3\frac{1}{5} \cdot 2.4$ **c.** $1\frac{7}{8} \cdot 2.4$

    _____   _____   _____

4. Calculate.

    a. $1\frac{7}{8} \cdot \frac{8}{15}$ **b.** $3\frac{1}{5} \cdot \frac{5}{16}$ **c.** $\frac{5}{12} \cdot 2.4$

    _____   _____   _____

5. Use multiplication to write three more equations, each with a product of 1.

_____

_____

_____

2-5 Progress Check

Extra Practice

1. Represent the fraction $\frac{10}{16}$ in each of these ways.

   a. An equivalent fraction in simplest form

   _____

   b. A position on the number line

   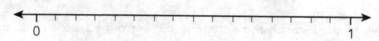

   c. The shaded part of a unit square

   d. A repeated addition

   _____

   e. A sum of two fractions with common denominators

   _____

   f. A sum of two fractions with different denominators

   _____

   g. A product of a whole number and a fraction

   _____

   h. A product of two fractions

   _____

Extra Practice continued _____

2. Represent the number $\frac{1}{1}$ in each of these ways.

a. An equivalent fraction _____

b. A repeated addition _____

c. A sum of two fractions with common denominators _____

d. A sum of two fractions with different denominators _____

e. A product of a whole number and a fraction _____

f. A product of two fractions _____

g. Using only variables _____

3. What advice would you give to a student who performed these calculations?

$$\frac{5}{8} + \frac{7}{24} = \frac{(5 \cdot 24) + (7 \cdot 8)}{8 \cdot 24} = \frac{120 + 56}{192} = \frac{176}{192}$$

$$\frac{5}{16} + \frac{3}{16} = \frac{(5 \cdot 16) + (3 \cdot 16)}{16 \cdot 16} = \frac{80 + 48}{256} = \frac{128}{256}$$

_____

_____

_____

_____

_____

2-6 Finding Differences

Extra Practice

1. Explain why each equation or inequality is true.

   a. $\frac{8}{12} - \frac{9}{12} = \frac{-1}{12}$

   _____

   _____

   b. $\frac{8}{12} = \frac{2}{3}$

   _____

   c. $\frac{9}{12} = \frac{3}{4}$

   _____

   d. $\frac{2}{3} < \frac{3}{4}$

   _____

2. **a.** Lisa calculated $\frac{11}{6} - \frac{7}{6}$ as $\frac{66}{36} - \frac{42}{36} = \frac{24}{36}$. Is the answer correct?

   _____

   b. What advice would you give to Lisa?

   _____

   _____

   _____

Extra Practice continued

3. a. Chen calculated $\frac{11}{20} - \frac{7}{30}$ as $\frac{11 \cdot 30}{20 \cdot 30} - \frac{7 \cdot 20}{30 \cdot 20} = \frac{330 - 140}{600} = \frac{190}{600}$. Is this correct?

_____

b. What advice would you give to Chen?

_____

_____

4. a. Rosa calculated $\frac{12}{20} - \frac{15}{30}$ as $\frac{12 \cdot 30}{20 \cdot 30} - \frac{15 \cdot 20}{30 \cdot 20} = \frac{360 - 300}{600} = \frac{60}{600}$. Is this correct?

_____

b. What advice would you give to Rosa?

_____

_____

_____

5. Annie, Lisa's sister, said that $\frac{7}{8} + \frac{7}{8} = \frac{14}{16}$. What advice would you give to Annie?

_____

_____

2-7 Addition and Subtraction as Inverses

Extra Practice

1. a. Perform the calculations to show that $1\frac{1}{4} - \frac{2}{5} = \frac{1}{10} + \frac{3}{4}$.

_____

_____

b. Perform the calculations to show that $\frac{2}{5} + \frac{1}{10} + \frac{3}{4} = 1\frac{1}{4}$.

_____

_____

c. Perform the calculations to show that $1\frac{1}{4} - \frac{2}{5} - \frac{1}{10} = \frac{3}{4}$.

_____

_____

d. Perform the calculations to show that $\frac{2}{5} = 1\frac{1}{4} - \frac{1}{10} - \frac{3}{4}$.

_____

_____

2. a. Sketch a number line of the equation $\frac{1}{2} + \frac{1}{3} + \frac{1}{4}$.

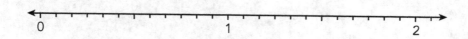

b. What scale did you use on your number line? _____

Extra Practice continued

3. Fill in the missing numbers in the square below.

The rule is that the following twelve sums must be the same:

- The sum of the five numbers in any row (↔)
- The sum of the five numbers in any column (↕)
- The sum of the five numbers along each of the two diagonals (↗ and ↘)

$\frac{19}{16}$	$\frac{7}{16}$	$\frac{5}{4}$	$\frac{13}{16}$	$\frac{1}{16}$
$\frac{5}{8}$	$\frac{3}{16}$	1	$\frac{9}{16}$	
$\frac{3}{8}$				
	$\frac{15}{16}$	$\frac{1}{2}$	$\frac{21}{16}$	
$\frac{23}{16}$			$\frac{17}{16}$	$\frac{5}{16}$

2-8   Shortest Distance

Extra Practice

1. Find the value of each equation when $a = \frac{3}{4}$, $b = \frac{1}{4}$, and $c = \frac{2}{3}$.

a. $a + b = \square$

b. $a + b + c = \square$

_____

_____

c. $a - b = \square$

d. $a - b + c = \square$

_____

_____

e. $ab = \square$

f. $\frac{a}{b} = \square$

_____

_____

g. $a - c = \square$

h. $b + c = \square$

_____

_____

i. $a \div b \div c = \square$

j. $ac = \square$

_____

_____

2. a. What conditions make the equation $\frac{a}{b} = 1$ true?

_____

b. What conditions make the equation $ab = 0$ true?

_____

Name _____ Class _____ Date_____

Extra Practice continued

3. Use the diagram and chart to answer the following questions about distances.

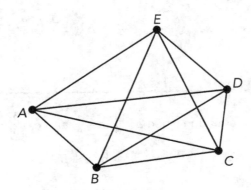

The following table shows the measure of the length of each line segment to the nearest sixteenth of an inch.

Segment	$\overline{AB}$	$\overline{AC}$	$\overline{AD}$	$\overline{AE}$	$\overline{BC}$
Length (in.)	$\frac{7}{8}$	2	2	$1\frac{1}{2}$	$1\frac{1}{4}$

Segment	$\overline{BD}$	$\overline{BE}$	$\overline{CD}$	$\overline{CE}$	$\overline{DE}$
Length (in.)	$1\frac{5}{8}$	$1\frac{9}{16}$	$\frac{9}{16}$	$1\frac{7}{16}$	$\frac{15}{16}$

a. Identify the four line segments that join the five points with the shortest possible total distance. What is the total distance?

_____

b. Find three paths from A to B that include one other point. What are the lengths of these paths? Which one is the shortest?

_____

_____

_____

c. What is the difference between the longest and shortest path listed in part (b)?

_____

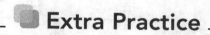

2-9 Dividing Fractions

Name _____ Class _____ Date _____

Extra Practice

1. Calculate the value of these expressions. Write your answers in simplest form.

a. $\frac{8}{5} \div \frac{4}{15}$

_____

b. $\frac{6}{5} \div \frac{3}{20}$

_____

c. $\frac{2}{3} \div \frac{3}{4}$

_____

d. $\frac{4}{15} \div \frac{8}{5}$

_____

e. $\frac{5}{6} \div \frac{20}{3}$

_____

f. $1\frac{3}{5} \div 2\frac{1}{2}$

_____

2. Check the answers to the previous problems by multiplying the answers by the original divisors.

a.

_____

b.

_____

c.

_____

d.

_____

e.

_____

f.

_____

Extra Practice continued _____

3. Rosa wrote $\frac{1}{10} \div \frac{3}{5} = \frac{1}{10} \cdot \frac{3}{5} = \frac{3}{50}$.

   a. What mistake did she make?

_____

_____

   b. What advice would you give Rosa?

_____

_____

_____

4. A cup holds $\frac{3}{8}$ liters of liquid when it is full.

   How many cups can you get from a bottle containing $2\frac{1}{4}$ liters?

_____

5. The gas mileage of a certain car is 30 miles per gallon.

   What is the mileage in kilometers per liter?

   (5 miles ≈ 8 kilometers, and $3\frac{3}{4}$ liters ≈ 1 gallon)

_____

2-10 Mixed Operations

Extra Practice

Use fractions to provide examples that show the following number properties.

1. An equation involving repeated addition can be written as a whole number multiplied by another number.

_____

2. $(a - b) - c = a - (b + c)$

_____

_____

3. $(a \div b) \div c = a \div bc$

_____

_____

4. $a(b + c) = ab + ac$

_____

_____

Extra Practice continued

5. $(a - b) \div c = (a \div c) - (b \div c)$

_____

_____

6. The product of a number and the reciprocal of the number is 1.

_____

7. A fraction with a denominator less than 10 can be written as an equivalent fraction with a denominator greater than 10.

_____

8. The average of two numbers is greater than one of the given numbers and less than the other.

_____

_____

Name _____ Class _____ Date _____

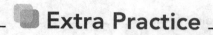

Progress Check

■ Extra Practice

1. Calculate.

   a. $\dfrac{7}{8} + \dfrac{7}{8} =$

   _____

   b. $\dfrac{7}{3} + \dfrac{3}{8} =$

   _____

   c. $\dfrac{7}{3} - \dfrac{5}{6} =$

   _____

   d. $2\dfrac{3}{5} + 1\dfrac{3}{4} =$

   _____

2. **a.** Sketch an area diagram to represent the calculation of $\dfrac{4}{3} \cdot \dfrac{5}{2}$.

   b. Explain how the answer is represented on the diagram.

   _____

   _____

   _____

   c. Write the equations involving division that are represented on the diagram.

   _____

Extra Practice continued

3. **a.** Calculate $\frac{4}{9} \cdot 2\frac{1}{4}$, and express the answer in simplest form. _____

   b. What is the reciprocal of $\frac{4}{7}$? _____

   c. Calculate $1 \div 1\frac{3}{7}$. _____

4. Calculate $\frac{9}{20}\left(\frac{4}{3} \cdot \frac{5}{2}\right)$, and express the answer in simplest form. _____

5. Which of these fractions is equal to $\frac{4}{9} \div \frac{7}{3}$?

   Ⓐ $\frac{28}{27}$ Ⓑ $\frac{63}{12}$ Ⓒ $\frac{27}{28}$ Ⓓ $\frac{12}{63}$

6. **a.** Calculate $\frac{5}{3}\left(\frac{3}{2} + \frac{3}{4}\right)$. _____

   b. Calculate $\left(\frac{5}{3} \cdot \frac{3}{2}\right) + \left(\frac{5}{3} \cdot \frac{3}{4}\right)$. _____

   c. Which number property explains why your answers to part (a) and part (b) should be the same?

_____

2-12 Shortest Time

Extra Practice

1. Keesha has four 2-hour DVDs and she wants to use them to record ten TV programs. The length of each program (in hours) is given in the table.

   Can she do it without using different DVDs for parts of the same program?

   If she can, explain how.

Program	Length (hours)	Program	Length (hours)
Presidential speech	$\frac{1}{6}$	Reality show	$\frac{2}{3}$
Variety program	$\frac{5}{6}$	Comedy	$\frac{1}{2}$
Cartoon	$\frac{1}{6}$	Local news	$\frac{1}{2}$
Fantasy adventure	$1\frac{11}{12}$	Thriller	$\frac{1}{2}$
Music program	$\frac{2}{3}$	Adventure	$1\frac{5}{6}$

DVDs

2 hrs   2 hrs   2 hrs   2 hrs

_____

_____

_____

_____

Extra Practice continued

2. The diagram shows the driving time in hours along the major highways that connect five California cities.

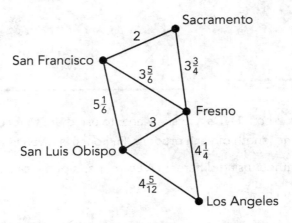

a. A sales representative based in Sacramento must visit the five cities for one day each and then drive back home. Which path involves the shortest driving time? Calculate the driving time for this path.

_____

_____

_____

b. Suppose the sales representative must visit Fresno and San Luis Obispo on consecutive days. Describe a route the sales representative could take. How much additional driving time would be involved compared to the route in part (a)?

_____

_____

_____

2-13 The Unit in Review

Extra Practice

1. $\frac{5}{16} + \frac{5}{16} =$

Ⓐ $\frac{10}{32}$ Ⓑ $\frac{5}{8}$ Ⓒ $\frac{5}{32}$ Ⓓ $\frac{5}{16}$

2. $3 \cdot \frac{4}{5} =$

Ⓐ $3\frac{4}{5}$ Ⓑ $\frac{12}{15}$ Ⓒ $\frac{12}{5}$ Ⓓ $\frac{4}{15}$

3. The equation $\frac{3}{4} \cdot \frac{7}{8} = \frac{21}{32}$ is equivalent to:

Ⓐ $\frac{21}{32} \div \frac{4}{3} = \frac{7}{8}$ Ⓑ $\frac{21}{32} \div \frac{7}{8} = \frac{3}{4}$ Ⓒ $\frac{3}{4} \div \frac{21}{32} = \frac{7}{8}$ Ⓓ $\frac{4}{3} \div \frac{7}{8} = \frac{21}{32}$

4. $\frac{5}{7} - \frac{2}{3} =$

Ⓐ $\frac{1}{21}$ Ⓑ $\frac{3}{4}$ Ⓒ $\frac{29}{21}$ Ⓓ $\frac{1}{7}$

5. $\frac{2}{7} + \frac{2}{7} + \frac{2}{7} + \frac{2}{7} + \frac{2}{7} + \frac{2}{7} + \frac{2}{7} =$

Ⓐ 7 Ⓑ $\frac{2}{49}$ Ⓒ $\frac{14}{49}$ Ⓓ 2

Extra Practice continued

6. In simplest form, $\frac{2}{5} \cdot \frac{3}{8} =$

  Ⓐ $\frac{31}{40}$ Ⓑ $\frac{6}{40}$ Ⓒ $1\frac{1}{15}$ Ⓓ $\frac{3}{20}$

7. $\frac{3}{7} \div \frac{5}{14} =$

  Ⓐ $\frac{6}{5}$ Ⓑ $\frac{15}{98}$ Ⓒ $\frac{5}{6}$ Ⓓ $\frac{11}{14}$

8. $2\frac{3}{8} \cdot \frac{3}{4} =$

  Ⓐ $\frac{6}{8} \cdot \frac{3}{4}$ Ⓑ $\left(2 \cdot \frac{3}{8}\right) + \left(2 \cdot \frac{3}{4}\right)$ Ⓒ $\left(2 \cdot \frac{3}{4}\right) + \left(\frac{3}{8} \cdot \frac{3}{4}\right)$ Ⓓ $2\left(\frac{3}{8} + \frac{3}{4}\right)$

9. $1\frac{2}{3} \div \frac{5}{3} =$

  Ⓐ 0 Ⓑ $\frac{9}{25}$ Ⓒ 1 Ⓓ $\frac{25}{9}$

3-1 Extending the Number Line

Extra Practice

1. When you write 3, do you mean +3 (positive 3) or −3 (negative 3)? _____

2. What is the value of each point on the following number lines?

a.
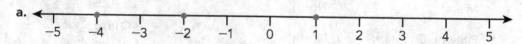

_____

b.
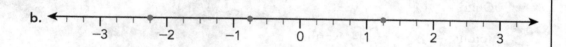

_____

c.
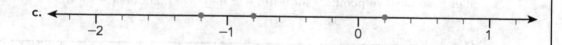

_____

d.
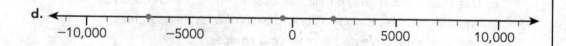

_____

e.
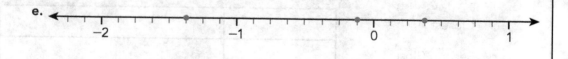

_____

Extra Practice continued

3. Lines of latitude run parallel to the equator. The latitude of the equator is 0°.

Every city in the world has a latitude, which is the number of degrees, north or south, of the equator.

This table lists the latitudes of some cities in North and South America:

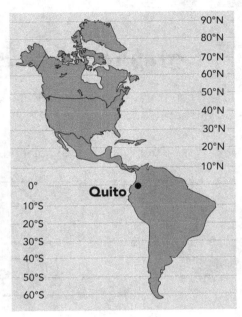

City	Latitude
Cape Horn	62° South
Lima	12° South
Miami	26° North
Panama City	9° North
Pittsburgh	41° North
Quito	0°
Toronto	44° North

a. Use the number line below to mark and label the point for each of the cities. Use positive numbers for north and negative numbers for south.

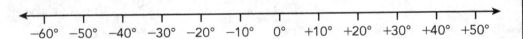

b. Use your number line to help you determine the difference in degrees of latitude between Panama City and each of the other six cities. Fill in your answers in the table and explain your choices.

Distance from Panama City	City	Explanation
Closest		
Second Closest		
Third Closest		
Fourth Closest		
Farthest		

3-2   Putting Numbers in Order

Extra Practice

1. Use the number lines for the following.

- On each number line, write the value of each labeled point.

- On the space provided below each number line, use *less than* symbols (<) between the numbers written in ascending order, from least to greatest.

a.
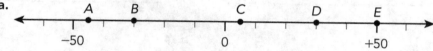

_____

b.
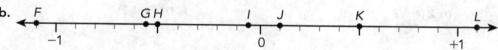

_____

c.
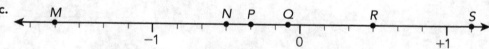

_____

d.
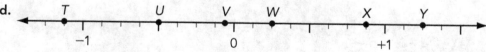

_____

Extra Practice continued

2. Label some points and a scale on the number line below. Then use *greater than* symbols (>) between the numbers written in descending order, from greatest to least.

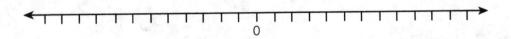

0

_____

3. Decide whether the following statements are true or false.

a. $-7 > -6$

b. $-3 < 9$

_____   _____

c. $-2\frac{1}{4} > -2$

d. $4 < -8$

_____   _____

e. $2 > -2$

f. $0 > -1.5$

_____   _____

g. $-3.1 < -3.01$

h. $6\frac{1}{2} \le -6\frac{1}{2}$

_____   _____

i. $-2.1 \le -2\frac{1}{10}$

j. $-5.2 < -4.6$

_____   _____

3-3 Adding with Negative Numbers

Extra Practice

1. Some students are playing a game that uses a number line and a stack of cards with positive and negative numbers on them. The rules are as follows.

- Lay the cards face down.

- Start at zero, and at each turn, flip over a card, and add the number it shows.

- The loser is the first person whose score goes outside the range −7 to +7.

  a. The first two numbers to come up are −1 and +3. On the number line, use arrows to illustrate the addition of these first two numbers. Remember to start at zero.

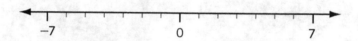

  b. Write the equation that is represented by the situation and calculate.

  _____

  c. The next number to come up is −4. Write the new equation and calculate.

  _____

  d. Here are the next numbers. Continue adding until the game ends.

  $$-2 \quad -1 \quad +3 \quad -4 \quad -2$$

  Write the equation for the step that lost the game and calculate.

  _____

Extra Practice continued _____

    e. Use your number line to calculate

       $(-1) + (+3) + (-4) + (-2) + (-1) + (+3) + (-4) + (-2) =$ _____

    f. Calculate $(-1) + (-4) + (-2) + (-1) + (-4) + (-2) + 3 + 3 =$ _____

    g. Explain why the answers to part (e) and part (f) should be the same.

    _____

    _____

    _____

2. Calculate.

    a. $(-5) + 8 =$ **b.** $(-8) + 5 =$

    _____   _____

    c. $4 + (-5) + 6 =$ **d.** $(-4) + 5 + (-6) =$

    _____   _____

    e. $(-2.3) + (-0.9) =$ **f.** $(-2.3) + 0.9 =$

    _____   _____

3-4 Subtracting with Negative Numbers

Extra Practice

1. Some students are playing a game that uses a number line and a stack of cards with positive and negative numbers on them. The rules are as follows.

- Lay the cards face down.

- Start at zero, and at each turn, flip over a card, and subtract the number it shows.

- The loser is the first person whose score goes outside the range −7 to +7.

   a. The first number turned over is +1, and the second number is −3.

   Remember that the rules are to start at zero and subtract each of the numbers.

   What number do the students calculate?

   _____

   b. The next number turned over is +4.

   Write the new equation and calculate.

   _____

2. Write the equation for the following number line and calculate.

_____

Extra Practice continued

3. Using the number lines below, sketch the difference, including direction, for each of the following calculations.

   a. $(-3) - 4 =$

   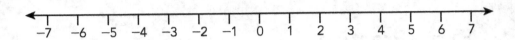

   b. $(-5) - (-3) =$

   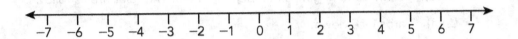

4. Calculate.

   a. $(-5) - 8 =$ b. $(-8) - 5 =$

   _____   _____

   c. $(-4) - (-5) =$ d. $(-6) - (-5) - (-4) =$

   _____   _____

   e. $(-5) - (-8) =$ f. $3 - (-4 + 5 - 6) =$

   _____   _____

   g. $(-2.2) + (-1.9) =$ h. $(-2.2) - (-1.9) =$

   _____   _____

3-5 Adding and Subtracting

Extra Practice

1. Convert the following to expressions involving addition, and evaluate.

    a. $230 - (-7) =$ **b.** $(-230) - (-17) =$

    _____   _____

    c. $(-230) - (-27) =$ **d.** $(-230) - (-7) =$

    _____   _____

2. Convert the following to expressions involving subtraction, and evaluate.

    a. $230 + (-7) =$ **b.** $(-230) + (-17) =$

    _____   _____

    c. $(-230) + (-27) =$ **d.** $(-230) + (-7) =$

    _____   _____

3. Calculate.

    a. $15.2 - (-16.15) =$ **b.** $(-8.04) - (-5.567) =$

    _____   _____

    c. $(-10.2) - (-20.18) =$ **d.** $7.8 + (-2.3) =$

    _____   _____

Extra Practice continued

4. a. Make up word problems that involve addition and subtraction of negative numbers.

_____

_____

_____

_____

_____

_____

b. Calculate your answers to these problems.

_____

_____

_____

_____

c. Write a short report on your solution methods and how to avoid errors.

_____

_____

_____

_____

_____

Name _____ Class _____ Date _____

3-6 Balloon Model

 Extra Practice

The height of an imaginary balloon above (positive) or below (negative) its normal operating height is influenced by:

- Weights: Each 1-unit change in weight moves the balloon up (losing weight) or down (gaining weight) by 1 meter.

- Hot air: Each 1-unit change in the amount of hot air in the balloon moves the balloon up (gaining hot air) or down (losing hot air) by 1 meter.

- Whether weight or hot air is *added* to the balloon, or *taken away* (subtracted) from the balloon.

On a vertical number line, 0 represents the normal operating height of the balloon.

Write equations to match each of the following stories based on the balloon model.

1. The balloon starts at a height of 8 meters below its normal operating height. 5 units of hot air are added into the balloon.

   To what height does the balloon move?

   _____

2. The balloon starts at a height of 5 meters below its normal operating height. 15 units of weight are then thrown (taken away) from the balloon.

   To what height does the balloon move?

   _____

Extra Practice continued

3. The balloon starts at a height of 8 meters above its normal operating height. 12 units of weight are then added to the balloon.

   To what height does the balloon move?

   _____

4. The balloon starts at a height of 6 meters below its normal operating height. 18 units of hot air are then released (taken away) from the balloon.

   To what height does the balloon move?

   _____

5. The balloon starts at a height of 6 meters above its normal operating height. 4 units of hot air and 7 units of weight are then released (taken away) from the balloon.

   To what height does the balloon move?

   _____

6. The balloon starts at a height of 9 meters above its normal operating height. 8 units of hot air are then released (taken away) from the balloon, and 12 units of weight are added.

   To what height does the balloon move?

   _____

7. The balloon starts at a height of 15 meters below its normal operating height. The release (taking away) of 3 units of hot air is repeated 5 times, and then 9 units of weight are added.

   What is the height of the balloon at the end?

   _____

3-7 Reviewing Addition and Subtraction

Extra Practice

1. Decide whether the following statements are true or false. Say why.

a. Negative 5 is less than negative 2.

_____

_____

b. $4 < 4$

_____

_____

c. $-3 \geq -3$

_____

_____

d. Negative 2 is less than positive 2.

_____

_____

e. Negative 100 is less than or equal to negative 1.

_____

_____

f. $0.50 > 0.5$

_____

_____

Extra Practice continued _____

g. $0.3333 \geq \frac{1}{3}$

_____

_____

h. $(-5.5) - (-8.5) = 5.5 - 8.5$

_____

_____

i. $(-3) + (-5) = (-3) - 5$

_____

_____

j. $(-8) - (-5) = (-5) - (-8)$

_____

_____

k. $(-7) + 6 = 6 + (-7)$

_____

_____

2. Calculate.

a. $245 - 15 =$ b. $225 + 15 =$ c. $(-300) - 5 =$ d. $(-300) + (-5) =$

_____   _____   _____   _____

e. $300 - 5 =$ f. $300 + (-5) =$ g. $450 - (-50) =$ h. $450 + 50 =$

_____   _____   _____   _____

i. $25 + 4.5 - 2.5 - (-2) =$ j. $5 + (-5) + 6 + (-12) + 6 =$

_____   _____

3-8 Multiplying and Dividing

Extra Practice

1.

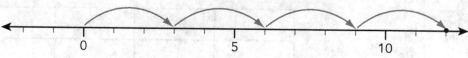

   a. Write a repeated addition equation to match the number line.

   _____

   b. Write your repeated addition equation as a multiplication equation.

   _____

2.

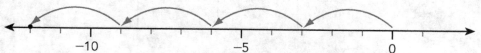

   a. Write a repeated addition equation to match the number line.

   _____

   b. Write your repeated addition equation as a multiplication equation.

   _____

3. Calculate.

   a. $(-6) \cdot 9 =$

   _____

   b. $8(-7) =$

   _____

   c. $\left(-\frac{3}{4}\right)\left(-\frac{4}{5}\right) =$

   _____

   d. $\left(-\frac{3}{4}\right)\left(\frac{4}{5}\right) =$

   _____

   e. $0.25(-0.8)$

   _____

   f. $0.24 \div (-0.8)$

   _____

Extra Practice continued

4. a. Fill in the cells of the table by performing the operation shown at the top of each column. Use the values for *a* and *b* that are given in each row. The first row has been done for you.

Use the completed table to answer parts (b) through (e).

a	b	a + b	a − b	ab	a ÷ b
6	−3	3	9	−18	−2
−6	3				
3	−6				
−3	6				
6	3				
−6	−3				
3	6				
−3	−6				

b. For which pairs of values of *a* and *b* does *ab* equal a negative number?

_____

c. What do the pairs of values that you listed in part (b) have in common?

_____

d. For which pairs of values of *a* and *b* does *a* ÷ *b* equal a positive number?

_____

e. What do the pairs of values that you listed in part (d) have in common?

_____

3-9 Order of Operations

Extra Practice

1. Calculate the value of each expression.

a. $32 \div 10 - 2$

_____

b. $32 \div (10 - 2)$

_____

c. $(25 + 8) \div 3 - 5 \cdot 3$

_____

d. $77 \div (11 - 4) \cdot 13$

_____

e. $20 + 5 \cdot 3$

_____

f. $(20 + 5) \cdot 3$

_____

g. $15 - (24 \div 6) + 3 \cdot 2$

_____

h. $43 - 39 \div 3 + 7$

_____

i. $196 \div 14 \cdot 3$

_____

j. $196 \div (14 \cdot 3)$

_____

k. $\dfrac{3^3}{11 - 5}$

_____

l. $\left(\dfrac{3}{11 - 5}\right)^3$

_____

Name _____ Class _____ Date _____

Extra Practice continued

2. Evaluate each expression for the given values of the variables.

a. $x - yz$ when $x = 2$, $y = 5$, and $z = 2$ _____

b. $a^2 - b - c$ when $a = 6$, $b = 4$, and $c = 1$ _____

c. $m(n - 1) + n^2$ when $m = 3$ and $n = 8$ _____

d. $ab - a(c - 3)$ when $a = 3$, $b = 12$, $c = 3$ _____

e. $x - y(10 - z)^2$ when $x = 50$, $y = 1$, $z = 8$ _____

f. $a \div bc$ when $a = -12$, $b = 3$, $c = 2$ _____

g. $a \div (bc)$ when $a = -12$, $b = 3$, $c = 2$ _____

h. $\frac{m^2}{n - p}$ when $m = -6$, $n = 11$, $p = 9$ _____

3-10 Mixed Operations

 Extra Practice

1. Calculate.

a. $-3 + [8 - (-12)] =$

_____

b. $(-3) + 8 - (-12) =$

_____

c. $-6 - (-8 + -4) =$

_____

d. $(-6) - (-8) + (-4) =$

_____

e. $(-12) \div [(-9)(-4)] =$

_____

f. $[(-12) \div (-9)](-4) =$

_____

g. $-10(-5 \cdot -2) =$

_____

h. $[(-10)(-5)] - [(-10) \cdot 2] =$

_____

i. $[(-32) \div (-8)] \div (-4)$

_____

j. $(-32) \div [(-8) \div (-4)]$

_____

k. $-9[(-3) + (-4)] =$

_____

l. $(-9)(-3) + (-9)(-4) =$

_____

Extra Practice continued

2. Calculate.

a. $(-0.3) + [0.8 - (-1.2)] =$ **b.** $-0.3 + 0.8 - (-1.2) =$

_____   _____

c. $(-0.6) - [(-0.08) + (-0.4)] =$ **d.** $-0.6 - (-0.08) + (-0.4) =$

_____   _____

e. $(-1.2) \div [(-0.9)(-0.4)] =$ **f.** $[(-1.2) \div (-0.9)](-0.4) =$

_____   _____

g. $(-10)[(-0.9) - 0.11] =$ **h.** $[-10(-0.9)] - [(-10) \cdot 0.11] =$

_____   _____

i. $[(-3.2) \div (-0.8)] \div (-0.4)$ **j.** $(-3.2) \div [(-0.8) \div (-0.4)]$

_____   _____

k. $-0.9[(-0.3) + (-0.4)] =$ **l.** $(-0.9)(-0.3) + (-0.9)(-0.4) =$

_____   _____

3. Make up some similar problems and calculate the answers.

_____

_____

_____

3-11 Number Properties

Extra Practice

1. Calculate the value of the following pairs of expressions.

   a. $(-5) - 8$ and $8 - (-5)$

   _____

   b. $6 - (-7)$ and $(-7) - 6$

   _____

   c. $4 - 12$ and $12 - 4$

   _____

   d. $(-8) - (-20)$ and $(-20) - (-8)$

   _____

   e. Write a general equation using variables that show the relationship in each pair of expressions.

   _____

2. The Distributive Property for subtraction is $a(b - c) = ab - ac$.

   a. Do the calculations to show that it is true for $a = -7$, $b = -4$, and $c = 6$.

   _____

   _____

   b. Do the calculations to show that it is true for $a = -9$, $b = 4$, and $c = -6$.

   _____

   _____

   c. Do the calculations to show that it is true for $a = 8$, $b = -4$, and $c = 6$.

   _____

   _____

Extra Practice continued

3. Calculate.

a. $1(-2) =$

_____

b. $(-2)(-2) =$

_____

c. $(-2)(-2)(-2) =$

_____

d. $(-2)(-2)(-2)(-2) =$

_____

e. $(-2)(-2)(-2)(-2)(-2) =$

_____

f. $(-2)(-2)(-2)(-2)(-2)(-2) =$

_____

g. How does the number of factors determine the sign of the product in a multiplication calculation?

_____

_____

_____

h. The value of $1 \div (-3) \div (-3) \div (-3) \div (-3) \div (-3)$ is between which two integers?

_____

3-12 Progress Check

Extra Practice

1. Write the following using symbols, and then calculate.

a. Negative 5 multiplied by negative 8

_____

b. Negative 8 divided by negative 5

_____

c. Negative 5 divided by negative 8

_____

d. Negative 5 added to negative 8

_____

e. Negative 5 subtracted from negative 8

_____

f. Negative 8 subtracted from negative 5

_____

2. Write the following using symbols, and then calculate.

a. Positive 0.05 multiplied by negative 8

_____

b. Negative 8 divided by positive 0.05

_____

c. Positive 0.05 divided by negative 8

_____

d. Positive 0.05 added to negative 8

_____

e. Positive 0.05 subtracted from negative 8

_____

f. Negative 8 subtracted from positive 0.05

_____

Extra Practice continued

3. Write the following using symbols, and then calculate.

a. Positive $\frac{2}{3}$ multiplied by positive $\frac{4}{5}$

_____

b. Positive $\frac{2}{3}$ divided by positive $\frac{4}{5}$

_____

c. Positive $\frac{4}{5}$ divided by positive $\frac{2}{3}$

_____

d. Positive $\frac{4}{5}$ added to positive $\frac{2}{3}$

_____

e. Positive $\frac{4}{5}$ subtracted from positive $\frac{2}{3}$

_____

f. Positive $\frac{2}{3}$ subtracted from positive $\frac{4}{5}$

_____

4. Make up an example of two numbers, a and b, that meets all of these conditions.

- The sum, $a + b$, is a positive number.
- The difference, $a - b$, is a negative number.
- The product is a negative number.
- ab is closer to zero than b is to zero.

_____

_____

_____

3-13 Absolute Value

Extra Practice

1. Evaluate each expression.

   a. $|-0.5|$

   _____

   b. $|-5| + |-4|$

   _____

   c. $|(-2) \cdot (-3)|$

   _____

   d. $\left|\dfrac{3}{2}\right|$

   _____

   e. $|3| - |-4|$

   _____

   f. $|-8| \div |2|$

   _____

2. Solve each equation.

   a. $|x| = 3.7$

   _____

   b. $0 = |x|$

   _____

   c. $|y| = (2 \cdot 3) - 5$

   _____

   d. $|c| = \dfrac{5}{2}$

   _____

Extra Practice continued

3. Graph the inequality $|x| < 1$ on the number line below.

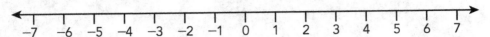

4. Graph the inequality $|x| > 1$ on the number line below.

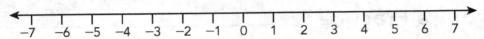

5. Summarize what you have learned about absolute value by completing this table.

$|x| = 1$	$|x| < 1$	$|x| > 1$
x = _____ or x = _____	x < _____ and x > _____	x > _____ or x < _____

6. Graph the inequality $|x| < 2.5$ on the number line below.

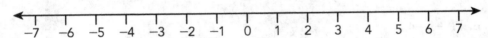

7. Graph the inequality $|x| > 2.5$ on the number line below.

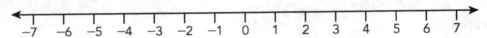

8. Summarize what you have learned about absolute value by completing this table.

$|x| = 2.5$	$|x| < 2.5$	$|x| > 2.5$
x = _____ or x = _____	x < _____ and x > _____	x > _____ or x < _____

It's Cold Up There

Extra Practice

In this problem, the temperature at ground level is 12°C. The temperature outside an airplane drops $2\frac{1}{2}$ degrees for every 1000 feet increase in the plane's height.

1. Complete this table.

Height (ft)	0	1000	3000	5000	10,000	20,000
Air Temperature (°C)						

Four students gave these answers when asked to sketch a graph of the relationship between the height of the airplane and the air temperature.

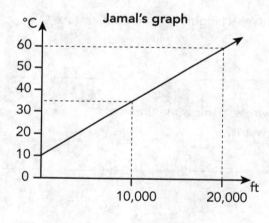

Jamal's graph

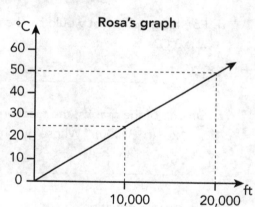

Rosa's graph

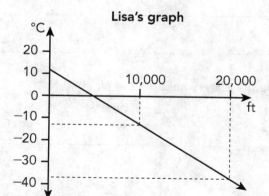

Lisa's graph

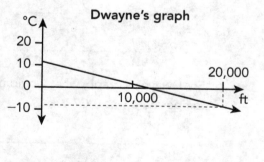

Dwayne's graph

Extra Practice continued

2. a. Which graph is the correct one? Say why.

_____

_____

b. On one of the graphs, the teacher wrote, "Well done! This is
$t = 12 - 2.5(h \div 1000)$." Whose graph was it?

_____

c. Explain the t, the h, and the equation.

_____

_____

_____

_____

d. For this graph, what would be the plane's height if the air temperature
was 0°C?

_____

e. On one of the graphs, the teacher wrote, "This is the graph of
$t = 12 - (h \div 1000)$." Whose graph was it?

_____

f. Explain the equation.

_____

_____

g. For Dwayne's graph, what would be the plane's height if the air
temperature was 0°C?

_____

3-15 Word Problems

Extra Practice

1. A student wrote $-10 > 1$.

   What possible misunderstandings could have led to this mistake?

   _____

   _____

2. A student wrote, "Negative 8 minus negative 20 is equal to 8 plus 20."

   What possible misunderstandings could have led to this mistake?

   _____

   _____

   _____

3. A student wrote $(-8)(-12) = -20$.

   What possible misunderstandings could have led to this mistake?

   _____

   _____

   _____

4. A student wrote $(-8) - 8 = 16$.

   What possible misunderstandings could have led to this mistake?

   _____

   _____

   _____

Extra Practice continued

5. A group of students were asked to calculate $(-8) - (-6 \cdot 4)$.

- One student wrote $-2 \cdot 4 = -8$.

- A second student wrote $-8 - (-24) = -32$.

- A third student wrote $-8 - (-24) = -16$.

What possible misunderstandings could have led to these mistakes?

_____

_____

_____

_____

_____

6. a. Calculate the value of $7 - 3x$ for $x = -6$. _____

b. Calculate the value of $3x - 7$ for $x = -6$. _____

c. Explain the relationship between part (a) and part (b).

_____

7. a. Calculate the value of $3x(3 - 2x)$ for $x = -4$. _____

b. Calculate the value of $9x - 6x^2$ for $x = -4$. _____

c. Explain the relationship between part (a) and part (b).

_____

3-16 The Unit in Review

Extra Practice

1. Use the following numbers: −6, 1.5, −0.75, −2, 3.

  a. Mark and label the numbers on the number line.

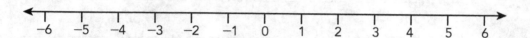

$$-6 \quad -5 \quad -4 \quad -3 \quad -2 \quad -1 \quad 0 \quad 1 \quad 2 \quad 3 \quad 4 \quad 5 \quad 6$$

  b. How many of the numbers are greater than 2? _____

  c. How many of the numbers are less than or equal to −2? _____

  d. Which two numbers are closest to each other on
  the number line? _____

2. Calculate.

  a. $4 + (−9) =$ **b.** $(−6) − (−17) =$ **c.** $(−3)(11) =$ **d.** $(−63) ÷ 9 =$

  _____   _____   _____   _____

  e. $(−18) − 4 + (−16) − (−5) =$ **f.** $(−10)(−6) − [8 ÷ (−2)]$

  _____   _____

3. Add parentheses to make these equations true.

  a. $8 ÷ 4 \cdot 2 + 1 = 2$

  b. $5 + (−7) \cdot (−4) − 3 − (−6) = −1$

Extra Practice continued

4. Decide whether the following statements are *always true, sometimes true,* or *never true.* Give examples to support your answers.

    a. If $a + b$ is a positive number, then either a or b must be a positive number.

    _____

    _____

    b. If ab is a positive number, then a and b are both positive numbers.

    _____

    _____

    c. If $a - b$ is a positive number, then b is greater than a.

    _____

    _____

5. Evaluate each expression.

    a. $|-27|$ **b.** $|-5| + |-3|$ **c.** $|(-4)(6)|$

    _____   _____   _____

6. Draw a number line for $|x| \geq 4$.

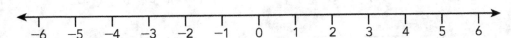

7. An amusement park ride requires a person to be within 6 inches of 42 inches tall. Use the equation $|h - 42| = 6$ to find the minimum and maximum heights for a person who wants to go on the ride.

_____

_____

4-1   Comparing Quantities

Extra Practice

1. Examine this set of squares and circles.

   a. Compare the number of squares to the number of circles using subtraction.

   _____

   _____

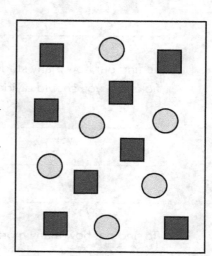

   b. Compare the number of squares to the number of circles using division.

   _____

   c. In the space at the right, sketch another set of squares and circles. In the new set, change the numbers of squares and circles, but keep the difference between the two numbers the same.

   d. Compare the ratio of squares to circles in your set to the ratio of squares to circles in the given set. Are they the same? Say why.

   _____

   _____

   _____

   _____

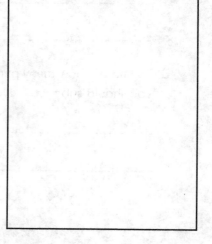

Extra Practice continued

2. Decide whether each statement is *true* or *false*. State which quantities should be subtracted or divided. Justify your answer.

a. To find out how many more boys than girls are in a class, you should divide.

_____

_____

_____

b. To find out how many students will ride on each bus for the ninth-grade field trip, you should divide.

_____

_____

_____

c. To find out how many more cats there are than dogs, you should subtract.

_____

_____

_____

d. To find out how many parking spaces there are for each store at a mall, you should subtract.

_____

_____

_____

Sample

To find out how much the temperature fell between 2 PM and 10 PM, you should subtract.

True. You would subtract the temperature at 10 PM from the temperature at 2 PM. Subtraction will give you the number of degrees the temperature fell.

4-2 Representing Ratios

Extra Practice

A music playlist contains 72 songs. There are 32 hip-hop songs and 40 rock songs.

1. Write the ratio of hip-hop songs to rock songs (a part-part comparison) as:

a. The simplest whole number ratio   **b.** A fraction in lowest terms

_____   _____

c. A decimal   **d.** A percent

_____   _____

2. Write the ratio of hip-hop songs to all the songs (a part-whole comparison) as:

a. The simplest whole number ratio   **b.** A fraction in lowest terms

_____   _____

c. A decimal (rounded to two decimal places)   **d.** A percent (rounded to the nearest whole percent)

_____   _____

3. The ratio 15 : 20 is equivalent to the ratio 3 : 4. Say why.

_____

_____

_____

Extra Practice continued

4. Express each of these ratios as a fraction in simplest form.

   a. 14 : 35   b. 15 : 18   c. 26 : 39

   _____   _____   _____

5. The fraction $\frac{2}{3}$ is equivalent to the ratio 2 : 3. Say why.

   _____

   _____

6. The number 0.4 is equivalent to the ratio 2 : 5. Say why.

   _____

   _____

7. 56% is equivalent to the ratio 14 : 25. Say why.

   _____

   _____

4-3 Unit Ratios and Equal Ratios

Extra Practice

1. A cooler at a picnic contains 20 lemon-lime drinks and 8 orange-mango drinks.

   a. Express the ratio of lemon-lime drinks to orange-mango drinks as the simplest whole number ratio. _____

   b. Explain what this ratio means.

      _____

      _____

   c. Express the ratio of lemon-lime drinks to orange-mango drinks as a unit ratio. _____

   d. Explain what this ratio means.

      _____

      _____

2. Jamal ate half of a sandwich, and Chen ate one-third.

   a. Write the simplest whole number ratio of the amount that Jamal ate to the amount that Chen ate. Justify your answer.

      _____

   b. Write the simplest whole number ratio of the amount that Chen ate to the amount that Jamal ate.

      _____

Extra Practice continued _____

3. Express each of these ratios as a unit ratio, rounded to three decimal places when necessary.

   a. 2 : 5

   _____

   b. 7 : 8

   _____

   c. 3.5 : 2.5

   _____

   d. $1\frac{1}{2} : 4\frac{1}{4}$

   _____

4. Express each of these ratios in simplest whole number form. Remember to first convert both quantities to the same unit.

   a. 50 cents to $2.50   _____

   b. 500 g to 12 kg   _____

   c. 3.2 km to 2400 m   _____

   d. 24 inches to 1 yard   _____

   e. 3 yards to 4 feet   _____

   f. 1000 cm to 1 m   _____

   g. 3 m to 1000 mm   _____

   h. 8 dimes to 4 nickels   _____

   i. 5 quarters to 1 dollar   _____

4-4 Ratio Tables

Extra Practice

1. a. Keesha wanted to invite 6 friends over to eat pizza and watch movies. She wanted to order 4 regular, uncut pizzas to share equally with her friends.

Complete this ratio table to show how much pizza there would be for each of the 7 people at Keesha's party.

Amount of Pizza	4	
Number of People	7	1

b. Chen was also having a pizza party. He invited 9 friends and wanted to order 5 regular, uncut pizzas.

Make a ratio table to show how much pizza there would be for each of the 10 people at Chen's party.

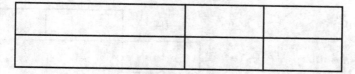

c. Which group of friends would get more pizza? Say how you know.

_____

_____

d. Keesha was surprised when 20 friends arrived at her house. She still wanted everyone to have the same ratio of pizza that she had originally planned. Extend your ratio table from 1(a) to find out how many pizzas Keesha needed to order for 20 friends.

_____

Extra Practice continued _____

2. Rosa's school is having a pancake breakfast to raise money for a class trip. Rosa is in charge of planning the food and beverages for the breakfast.

    a. Rosa finds a pancake recipe that requires 2 cups of flour to make 15 pancakes. Complete this ratio table to show how much flour is needed to make different numbers of pancakes.

Number of Pancakes	15	30	60	90
Cups of Flour	2			

    b. Rosa decides that they will make 150 pancakes at the breakfast. How much flour will be needed? Say how you know.

_____

_____

_____

_____

    c. Rosa plans to get large bottles of orange juice that each contain 128 fluid ounces of juice. Each bottle serves 16 people. Complete the ratio table.

Fluid Ounces of Juice	128	64		
Number of Servings	16		2	1

    d. Each bottle of juice costs $6. Rosa estimates that they will need 5, 6, or 7 bottles for the pancake breakfast. Make a ratio table to show how much it will cost to buy 5, 6, or 7 bottles of the juice.

4-5 Solving Proportion Problems with Ratio Tables

Extra Practice

1. Here are the ingredients to make 30 cookies. The quantities of ingredients needed to make any number of cookies are in proportion to these quantities.

2 cups of flour

$\frac{1}{2}$ teaspoon of vanilla

$\frac{1}{4}$ cup of milk

3 eggs

$\frac{1}{3}$ cup of butter

$\frac{3}{4}$ cup of sugar

a. Dwayne wants to make some cookies, but he has 5 eggs. What is the maximum number of cookies he could make, and what are the quantities of all the ingredients that he would need to make that number of cookies?

_____

_____

_____

b. Which measurements might Dwayne have to round up or down? Say why.

_____

_____

_____

_____

_____

_____

Extra Practice continued

c. Dwayne also considers making batches of 20, 60, and 40 cookies. To help Dwayne, complete this ratio table.

Number of Cookies	30	20	60	40
Cups of Flour				
Cups of Milk				
Cups of Butter				
Eggs				
Cups of Sugar				
Teaspoons of Vanilla				

2. a. Dwayne has a 2-pound (32-ounce) bag of flour. He looks in a cookbook and finds that 1 cup of flour weighs 4 ounces.

How many cups of flour are in Dwayne's bag of flour?

_____

b. Dwayne wants to use the whole bag of flour to make cookies. How many cookies can he make if he buys more eggs?

_____

c. How much of each ingredient will Dwayne need in order to make the number of cookies you calculated in 2(b)?

_____

_____

4-6 More About Solving Proportion Problems

◼ Extra Practice

1. Rosa and Lisa are practicing free throws on the basketball court. So far, Rosa has made one-and-a-half times as many free throws as Lisa.

   a. What is the unit ratio of Rosa's free throws to Lisa's free throws? _____

   b. What is the simplest whole number ratio? _____

   c. Rosa has made 18 free throws. Complete the ratio table to find the number of free throws that Lisa has made.

Rosa			18
Lisa	1	2	

2. a. At a pet rescue center, the ratio of cats to dogs is 3 : 5. There are 21 cats at the center. In the space below, draw a bar diagram that you can use to determine the number of dogs at the center.

   b. How many dogs are at the center? Say how you know.

   _____

   _____

   _____

Extra Practice continued

3. A group of people has a ratio of left-handers to right-handers of 2 : 7. If there are 14 right-handers, how many left-handers are in the group?

   In the space below, use a ratio table, a bar diagram, and an equation to solve the problem. Then write the answer on the line below.

   _____

4. Chen's mother manages a pharmacy. In the past two months, the pharmacy's revenue was $120,000 and expenses at the pharmacy were $85,000.

   Over the next twelve months, Mrs. Lee wants to keep this ratio (money received to money spent) constant. If expenses over the next twelve months are $95,000, how much money is needed in revenue?

   In the space below, use a ratio table and an equation to solve the problem. Then write the answer on the line below.

   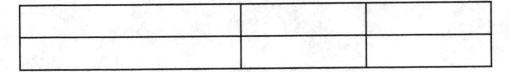

   _____

4-7 Introducing Rates

Extra Practice

1. A car traveled 300 miles in 5 hours.

    a. At what average speed (rate) did the car travel?

    _____

    b. At this rate, how far would the car travel in 6 hours?

    _____

    c. At this rate, how long would the car take to travel 480 miles?

    _____

2. Mrs. Jackson's bank pays interest on her savings at the rate of 5% per year. Interest is calculated and added to the balance at the end of the year.

    a. A rate of 5% per year is equivalent to a ratio of 1 : 20. Say why.

    _____

    b. Suppose Mrs. Jackson has $300 in the bank. How much interest will she earn in one year?   _____

    c. If Mrs. Jackson always leaves the interest in the bank, how much interest will she earn on the total at the end of the next year?   _____

    d. At the end of two years, how much money does Mrs. Jackson have in the bank?

    _____

    e. Suppose the rate of interest is halved (that is, cut in half). How much interest will she earn on $300 in one year?   _____

Extra Practice continued

3. A machine has two gear wheels that interconnect. The larger gear wheel has 10 teeth, and the smaller gear wheel has 6 teeth.

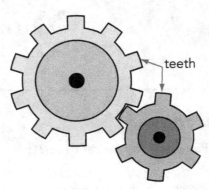

teeth

a. What is the unit ratio of the number of teeth on the large wheel to the number of teeth on the small wheel?

_____

b. When the larger wheel makes one complete turn, how many turns will the smaller wheel make?

_____

c. The rate at which the larger wheel turns is 20 revolutions (complete turns) per second. At what rate is the smaller wheel turning?

_____

d. If the smaller wheel turns 20 revolutions per second, at what rate is the larger wheel turning?

_____

4-8 Reviewing Ratio and Arithmetic

Extra Practice

Read each of the following statements and decide whether it is *always true*, *sometimes true*, or *never true*. Justify your answer for each statement. When possible, give examples, using numbers, to support your reasoning.

1. If you compare two numbers using division, you will get the same result that you would get if you compared the two numbers using subtraction.

   _____

   _____

   _____

2. You find a ratio by dividing one number by another number (except zero).

   _____

   _____

3. As a ratio of two quantities gets closer to equaling 1, the two quantities get closer to being the same.

   _____

   _____

4. A percent can be thought of as a ratio.

   _____

   _____

Extra Practice continued

5. If two quantities have units that are different, you can find the ratio of the quantities by converting one unit to the other.

_____

_____

6. A ratio table is a collection of equal ratios.

_____

_____

7. To find an unknown number using a ratio table, use the operation of multiplication.

_____

_____

8. A ratio of whole numbers can be expressed as a unit ratio.

_____

_____

9. Any whole number ratio can be converted to a unit ratio.

_____

_____

10. A rate is also a ratio.

_____

_____

4-9 Enlarging and Reducing

Extra Practice

1. A photograph has a width of 8 cm and a height of 12 cm.

   a. Calculate the unit ratio of width to height. _____

   b. What is the simplest whole number ratio of height to width? _____

2. A photo shop wants to reduce the photograph from Problem 1 so that the photo's height is $9\frac{1}{2}$ cm, as shown below.

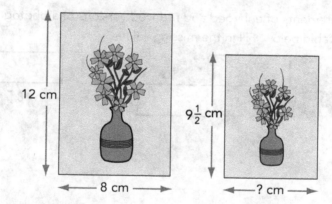

   a. What is the ratio of the width to the height? _____

   b. Use this ratio to find the width of the smaller photograph. _____

   c. What is the ratio of the height to the width? _____

   d. How can you use this ratio to find the width of the smaller photograph?

   _____

   _____

   _____

Extra Practice continued _____

3. Which of the following measurements represent an enlarged or reduced version of the photo in Problem 1?

   a. 8 cm wide by 10 cm high   _____

   b. 5 cm wide by 7.5 cm high   _____

   c. 13 cm wide by 17 cm high   _____

   d. 12 cm wide by 18 cm high   _____

   e. 7 cm wide by 10.5 cm high   _____

   f. 16.5 cm wide by 25 cm high   _____

   g. 18 cm wide by 24 cm high   _____

4. Some measurements of enlarged and reduced versions of a photograph are listed in the table below. Fill in the missing values.

Width (cm)		5	10		7.5
Height (cm)	3		12	18	

4-10 Scale Factor and Ratio

Extra Practice

1. A model car is constructed using a 1 : 20 scale. This model has a scale factor of $\frac{1}{20}$ in relation to the original car.

   a. Write the scale factor $\frac{1}{20}$ as a percent.   _____

   b. If the real car is 12 feet long, how long will the model be?   _____

   c. If the real car is 6 feet wide, how wide will the model be?   _____

   d. If the model is 0.25 feet tall, how tall is the real car?   _____

2. Lisa wants to enlarge a photo that has a width of 8 cm and a height of 12 cm so that the photo will have a width of 20 cm.

   a. What is the scale factor of the enlargement?   _____

   b. What will the height of the new photo be?   _____

   c. Next, Lisa decides to reduce the enlargement to produce a photo with the original dimensions. What scale factor should she use? Explain your answer.

   _____

   _____

Extra Practice continued _____

3. A photographer wants to print three copies of a photograph on the same sheet of paper—one larger version and two smaller ones. She decides to arrange them as shown in the diagram.

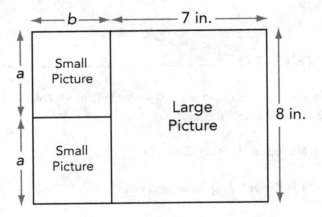

    a. What is the ratio between the width of the larger copy and the width of the smaller copies?

_____

    b. What are the missing measurements (*a* and *b*)?

_____

4-11 Unit Price

Extra Practice

Problems 1 and 2 refer to this table, which shows the rates charged by the Rapid Delivery Service company. Rapid Delivery Service charges by the weight of the package and the distance it needs to travel. The company has divided the distance into different zones. (Increasing zone numbers mean increasing distances.)

Zone	Economy Rate (per 1-lb package)	One-Day Rate (per 1-lb package)	Two-Day Rate (per 1-lb package)
1	$0.50	$0.75	$0.50
2	$0.50	$1.50	$0.75
3	$0.75	$2.25	$1.00
4	$1.25	$3.00	$2.00

1. The packages listed below were sent using the Economy Rate.

   a. Complete this table.

Weight of Package Sent to Zone 1 (pounds) w	5	10	15	20
Cost (dollars) c				

   b. In the space at the right, sketch a graph to represent the relationship between the weight of the packages and the cost for the Economy Rate to Zone 1.

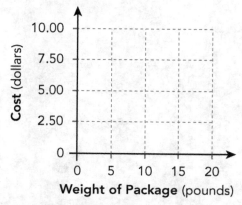

Extra Practice continued _____

c. Keesha's friend Zoe lives in Zone 1. Keesha sends her a package at the Economy Rate. The package weighs 3 pounds. How much will shipping the package cost Keesha? _____

d. Keesha sends another package to a different friend in Zone 1 using the Two-Day Rate. The cost to send the package is $5.50. How much did the package weigh? _____

e. The delivery service uses a minimum weight of 1 pound. What is the cost of a 1-pound package to Zone 3 at the One-Day Rate? _____

f. How much will Keesha pay to send a 27-pound package to Zoe (in Zone 1) at the Two-Day Rate? _____

g. Keesha sends a 27-pound package to Zoe (in Zone 1) at the One-Day Rate. Compare this cost with the cost of the package sent at the Two-Day Rate.

_____

2. Consider the table of Rapid Delivery Service charges again.

a. For which rate (Economy, One-Day, or Two-Day) does the cost increase by a constant amount for each increase in zone? _____

b. How much would Keesha be charged to send a 12-pound package to her friend Lizzie, who lives in Zone 4, at the One-Day Rate? _____

4-12 Unit Conversion

Extra Practice

1. There are 3.79 liters in one gallon. There are 0.254 gallons in one liter.

   a. How many liters of gasoline does a 26-gallon fuel tank hold?

   _____

   b. How many gallons of gasoline does a 500-liter fuel tank hold?

   _____

2. There are 16 ounces in one pound. There are 2.2 pounds in one kilogram.

   a. What is the conversion factor for kilograms to ounces?

   _____

   b. How many ounces are there in 3 kilograms?

   _____

   c. How many kilograms are there in 211.2 ounces?

   _____

3. There are 4 quarts in one gallon. There are 2 pints in one quart.

   a. What is the conversion factor for quarts to gallons?

   _____

   b. What is the conversion factor for pints to gallons?

   _____

   c. How many gallons are there in 72 pints?

   _____

Extra Practice continued

4. In this problem, "USD" means *American dollars*, and "AUD" means *Australian dollars*.

Suppose it costs USD 0.72 to buy AUD 1.

a. What is the conversion factor for Australian dollars to American dollars?

_____

b. How many American dollars can be bought with AUD 50?

_____

c. How many American dollars can be bought with AUD 180?

_____

d. What is the conversion factor for American dollars to Australian dollars?

_____

e. How many Australian dollars can be bought with USD 50?

_____

f. How many Australian dollars can be bought with USD 180?

_____

4-13 Unit Analysis

Extra Practice

1. Write the operation that you would need to achieve the unit $\frac{gallons}{mile}$ beginning with these given units. Explain your answers.

   a. *gallons* and *miles*

   _____

   b. $\frac{miles}{gallon}$

   _____

   c. $\frac{gallons}{hour}$ and $\frac{miles}{hour}$

   _____

2. This rectangle has a width of 5 meters and a length *l* also in meters.

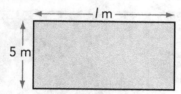

   Use unit analysis to calculate the rate (in square meters per minute) at which the area is increasing if the length is increasing at the rate of 0.5 meters per minute.

   _____

Extra Practice continued

3. Carlos is setting up a new aquarium. He attaches a hose to the kitchen faucet and finds that the hose adds 5 gallons of water to the aquarium every 2.5 minutes. Carlos knows that one gallon of water weighs 8.3 pounds. He wants to know the rate at which the weight of the aquarium is increasing.

   a. What are the units for the rates that are given in the problem?

   _____

   b. What is the unit for the rate that Carlos wants to find?

   _____

   c. What operation do you need to use to achieve the unit in 3(b)? Explain.

   _____

   d. At what rate is the weight of the aquarium increasing?

   _____

   e. It takes Carlos 12.5 minutes to fill the aquarium. What is the weight of the water in the aquarium when it is full?

   _____

Name _____ Class _____ Date _____

4-14 Representing Proportional Relationships

Extra Practice

Dwayne's aunt works for a company that manufactures and sells flags.

Dwayne's aunt is preparing all of the stripes for an order of a large quantify of flags. She wants to determine a rule so she knows how many stripes to prepare. She thinks about the relationship between the number of stripes (*S*) she will need in order to make a certain number of U.S. flags (*f*).

1. Name the quantities that are proportional to each other.

_____

2. Write the unit ratio for the number of stripes to the number of flags. (The U.S. flag has 13 stripes.)

_____

3. Express your answer to Problem 2 as a rate.

_____

4. What is the constant of proportionality in this relationship?

_____

5. Write a formula for the number of stripes *S* in terms of the number of flags *f*.

_____

Extra Practice continued

6. Sketch a graph of the number of stripes and the number of flags. Put the number of stripes on the vertical axis and mark the number of flags from 0 to 10 on the horizontal axis.

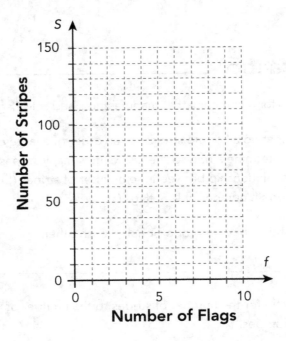

Number of Flags

7. If Dwayne's aunt needs to make 50 flags, how many stripes does she need? Show how you calculated your answer.

_____

8. How many flags can Dwayne's aunt make if she has prepared 585 stripes? Show how you calculated your answer.

_____

Name _____ Class _____ Date _____

Extra Practice

1. Each table below is a ratio table because there is a constant of proportionality k between each pair of values.

   For each table, calculate the constant of proportionality using $\frac{y}{x} = k$.

   (You may want to use a calculator.)

   a.   _____

x	y
4	2.4
5	3
7	4.2
12	7.2
17	10.2

   b.   _____

x	y
4	9
5	11.25
7	15.75
12	27
17	38.25

   c. Write a formula in the form of $y = kx$ for 1(a).   _____

   d. Write a formula in the form of $y = kx$ for 1(b).   _____

Name _____ Class _____ Date _____

Extra Practice continued

2. The graph below represents the relationship between the volume of sand in a container and the height of the sand.

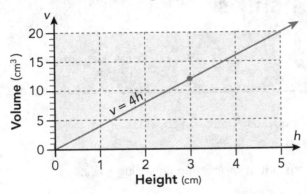
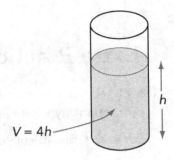

a. What does the point (3, 12) on the graph represent?

_____

_____

b. In this situation, the volume of sand is proportional to the height of the sand. Say why.

_____

_____

c. What is the constant of proportionality, and what does it represent in this situation?

_____

_____

d. Suppose you adjust the graph so that the total volume for the container is 100 cm^3. What would be the value for h?

_____

4-16 Graphing Proportional Relationships

Extra Practice

1. Imagine a hanging spring that is stretched by attaching weights to the bottom.

The length of the spring increases by 6 cm when a 1-gram weight is attached to it.

The length of the spring increases by 12 cm when a 2-gram weight is attached to it.

The length of the spring increases by 18 cm when a 3-gram weight is attached to it, and so on.

In this table, x represents the weight (in grams), and y represents the increase in length (in centimeters) when each weight is attached to the spring.

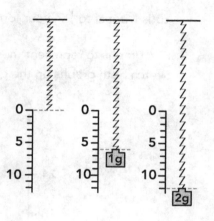

x (grams)	0	1	2	3	4	5
y (cm)	0	6	12	18	24	30

a. Is y proportional to x? _____

b. Write the formula that represents the relationship of y to x. _____

c. Is $\frac{y}{x}$ the same for every (x, y) pair in the table?

_____

d. Is k equal to $\frac{y}{x}$ in your formula? _____

Extra Practice continued

2. Repeat 1(a–d) for a second spring that increases in length by 4 cm for every 1-gram weight that is attached to it.

   a. Is y proportional to x?   _____

   b. Write the formula that represents the relationship of y to x.   _____

   c. Is $\frac{y}{x}$ the same for every (x, y) pair?

   _____

   d. Is k equal to $\frac{y}{x}$ in your formula?   _____

3. Plot graphs to represent the proportional relationships in Problems 1 and 2. Sketch both graphs on the grid below. Which graph is steeper? Say why.

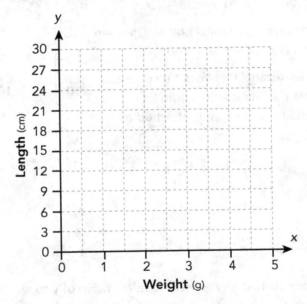

_____

_____

4-17 Formulas and Proportional Relationships

Extra Practice

1. A stack of 8 identical coins is 1.6 cm high. Show that this information satisfies the formula $n = 5h$, where n is the number of coins and h is the height of the stack in centimeters.

   _____

   _____

2. If you double the number of coins in a stack of identical coins, what happens to the height?

   _____

   _____

3. In the space below, make a table that relates the values of n and h for the formula $n = 5h$. Include entries for $h = 1$ to $h = 15$.

4. How many coins from Problem 1 would be in a stack 80 cm high?   _____

Extra Practice continued

5. The formula $n = 5h$ gives the number of coins in terms of the height of the stack. Write a formula for h in terms of n.

_____

6. The constant of proportionality in the formula in Problem 5 is the multiplicative inverse of the constant of proportionality in the formula in Problem 1. Say why.

_____

_____

7. Suppose there is another type of coin for which the formula for n in terms of h is $n = 4h$. Is this coin thicker or thinner than the first type (for which the formula is $n = 5h$)? Say why.

_____

_____

_____

Extra Practice

1. a. Use an arrow and words to represent each of these three functions.

$y = 50x$

$y = \frac{5}{6}x$

$y = 0.08x$

b. Complete these three tables of values—one for each of the three functions above. Use each function to calculate the y-values corresponding to the given x-values. (*Comment:* Students may use a calculator.)

x	1	0.5	10	35	367	10,200
y						

x	1	0.5	10	35	367	10,200
y						

x	1	0.5	10	35	367	10,200
y						

Extra Practice continued

2. Jamal's cousin Ameera is calculating the fuel efficiency of her car. According to Ameera, the car can travel 25 miles on one gallon of gasoline.

   a. Jamal thinks the number of miles m that the car can travel is a function of the number of gallons of gasoline g that the car uses.

   Do you agree with Jamal? Explain. Support your conclusion using an arrow and words, a table, a graph, and a formula.

   Arrow and words:

   Table:

   Graph:

   Formula and explanation:

   _____

   _____

   b. Jamal does not think that the number of gallons g is a function of the number of miles m.

   Do you agree with Jamal? Explain.

   _____

   _____

4-19 Inversely Proportional Relationships

■ Extra Practice

1. The chart below shows pictures, formulas, verbal descriptions, graphs, and tables for four functions.

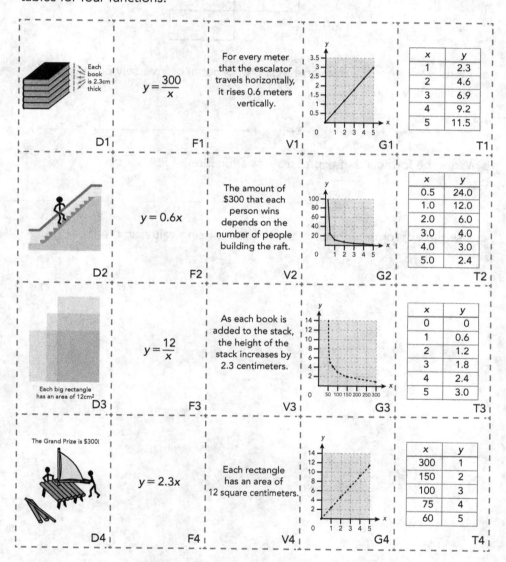

Each book is 2.3cm thick **D1**	$y = \dfrac{300}{x}$ **F1**	For every meter that the escalator travels horizontally, it rises 0.6 meters vertically. **V1**	*graph* **G1**	x y 1 2.3 2 4.6 3 6.9 4 9.2 5 11.5 **T1**
escalator picture **D2**	$y = 0.6x$ **F2**	The amount of $300 that each person wins depends on the number of people building the raft. **V2**	*graph* **G2**	x y 0.5 24.0 1.0 12.0 2.0 6.0 3.0 4.0 4.0 3.0 5.0 2.4 **T2**
Each big rectangle has an area of 12cm² **D3**	$y = \dfrac{12}{x}$ **F3**	As each book is added to the stack, the height of the stack increases by 2.3 centimeters. **V3**	*graph* **G3**	x y 0 0 1 0.6 2 1.2 3 1.8 4 2.4 5 3.0 **T3**
The Grand Prize is $300! **D4**	$y = 2.3x$ **F4**	Each rectangle has an area of 12 square centimeters. **V4**	*graph* **G4**	x y 300 1 150 2 100 3 75 4 60 5 **T4**

a. Find sets of one picture, one formula, one verbal description, one graph, and one table that represent the same function. Write the four sets below.

Set 1: _____   Set 2: _____

Set 3: _____   Set 4: _____

Extra Practice continued

    b. Which sets of representations are proportional relationships? Which are inversely proportional relationships?

_____

_____

2. Given this table of values:

x	0.3	4		10
y	4.5	60	72	

    a. Identify whether the relationship is proportional or inversely proportional, and say how you know.

_____

    b. Write the formula that expresses y as a function of x.

_____

    c. Use the appropriate function to fill in the missing values in the table.

Name _____ Class _____ Date _____

4-20 Distance, Ratio, and Proportionality

 Extra Practice _____

Lisa bought a new bicycle. She collected some data to compare how far the bicycle would travel in low gear and in high gear. These are her measurements.

Low Gear

Number of Turns of the Pedals	5	7	9
Distance Traveled (feet and inches)	30'10"	43'2"	55'6"

High Gear

Number of Turns of the Pedals	2	3	5
Distance Traveled (feet and inches)	37'	55'6"	92'6"

1. Lisa thinks the two variables are in proportional relationships in each situation, but she is not sure. Write an explanation that makes this clear for Lisa. (*Hint:* First convert the distances to feet, and express each as an improper fraction in lowest terms.)

   _____

   _____

   _____

2. What is the ratio of distance covered by one complete turn of the pedals for high gear to low gear?

   _____

3. If Lisa pedals the same number of times in high gear as in low gear, how many times farther does she travel in high gear?

   _____

Name _____ Class _____ Date _____

4. At what rate (feet per pedal turn) is Lisa traveling when she is in each gear?

_____

_____

5. Write two formulas (one for each gear) that will tell Lisa how far she will travel (*d* feet) if the pedals turn *t* times.

_____

6. Write two formulas (one for each gear) that will tell Lisa how many times the pedals will turn (*t*) if she travels *d* feet.

_____

7. Plot graphs of the formulas you found for Problem 6. Use the coordinate plane below for both graphs.

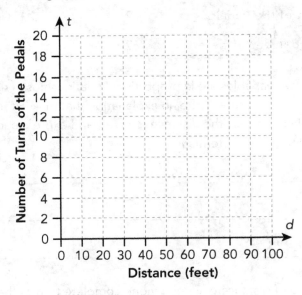

8. The library is 1850 feet away from Lisa's house. How many turns of the pedals would it take her to ride to the library in each gear?

_____

4-21 Geometry, Ratio, and Proportionality

Extra Practice

These problems refer to triangles that share the same base.

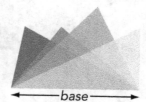

←—— base ——→

The triangles have the following properties:

- base = 14 centimeters
- height (in centimeters) = h
- Area (in square centimeters) = A

1. Express A in terms of h: that is, write a formula that uses A to represent the area and h to represent the height.

_____

2. Find the value of A for each of the following values of h.

   a. $h = 2.5$ cm   **b.** $h = 7.5$ cm   **c.** $h = 12.5$ cm

_____ _____ _____

3. Fill in the missing values in the table.

Height (cm)	1	4.5		11.5		h
Area (cm²)			70		112	

Name _____ Class _____ Date _____

Extra Practice continued _____

4. What is the constant of proportionality for the relationship? _____

5. What does the constant of proportionality represent in this situation?

_____

_____

6. Represent the relationship of *A* in terms of *h* by making a graph on the coordinate plane below.

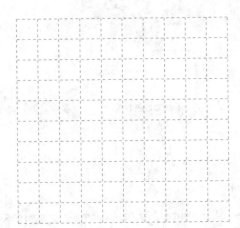

4-22 Mountain Trip

Extra Practice

1. A car is traveling at 40 miles per hour with an average fuel economy of 25 mpg.

   a. Complete the following table for this car.

Traveling Time (minutes) t	0	15	30	60	120
Fuel Used (gallons) f	0				
Fuel in Tank (gallons) $y = 20 - f$	20				

   b. Which of these three relationships, f to t, y to t, and y to f, are increasing relationships?

   _____

   c. Which one of these three relationships is a proportional relationship? What is its constant of proportionality?

   _____

   d. Which of these three variables could have a proportional relationship with the distance d traveled? Say why.

   _____

   _____

   _____

Extra Practice continued

2. Look for a pattern in the following table.

Height Above Sea Level (feet) h	4000	5000	6000	7000	8000	9000	10,000
Outside Air Temperature (°F) T	40.0	33.3	26.7	20.0	13.3	6.7	0.0

a. What pattern do you see in the table?

_____

_____

b. Is the relationship between the variables an increasing relationship or a decreasing relationship?

_____

c. Is the relationship between the variables a proportional relationship? Explain how your answer can be obtained by looking at the table.

_____

_____

_____

_____

4-23 The Unit in Review

🔲 Extra Practice

1. The diagram below shows the measurements made on one side of a river.

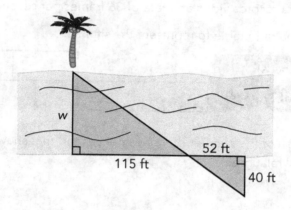

About how wide is the river? _____

2. a. What is the unit price for 1.5 kg of potatoes that cost $3.75? _____

b. What is the unit price for 3.5 kg of potatoes that cost $8.47? _____

c. What is the unit price for 5 kg of potatoes that cost $12.20? _____

d. Of the potatoes in 2(a–c), which is the best buy? Explain.

_____

_____

3. A path with constant steepness rises 280 feet in elevation over the first 0.8 km. How much does the path rise in elevation over its entire 2.5-km length?

_____

Extra Practice continued

4. If a computer enlarges a 3 in. × 4.5 in. photograph to a 7 in. × 10.5 in. photograph, then both images (large and small) will be in proportion. Say why.

_____

_____

_____

5. A certain camera records video at a rate of 36 frames per second.

   a. Complete the ratio table to represent the situation.

Time (seconds) t	1	3			20
Number of Frames f			180	270	

   b. Make a graph of the number of frames per second that shows the proportional relationship.

   c. Write two formulas: one for the number of frames in terms of time, and one for time in terms of the number of frames.

   _____

   d. Use one of your formulas to determine the number of frames the camera records during a 12-second video.

   _____

   _____

5-1 Building the Coordinate Plane

Extra Practice

1. Plot a point in each quadrant in the graph below.

   a. Represent each of your points with
      coordinates in the form (x, y).

     _____

   b. Identify the quadrant in which each of
      your points lies.

     _____

     _____

     _____

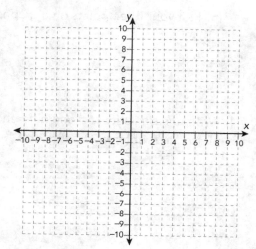

2. Choose an x-value.

   a. Represent three points in the form
      (x, y) using your x-value with different
      y-values. Choose at least one y-value
      that is negative and at least one
      y-value that is not an integer.

     _____

   b. Plot your three points on a graph.

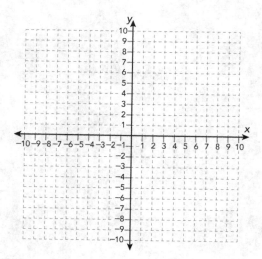

Extra Practice continued

3. Choose a *y*-value.

    a. Represent three points in the form (*x*, *y*) using your y-value with different *x*-values. Choose at least one *x*-value that is negative and at least one *x*-value that is not an integer.

    _____

    b. Plot your three points on a graph.

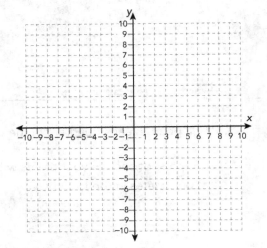

4. Write one similarity and one difference between the two sets of points you plotted in Problems 2(b) and 3(b).

_____

_____

_____

5-2 Constant Ratios and Graphing

● Extra Practice

1. Plot each point below on the coordinate plane.

    a. $(1.5, -1)$ **b.** $\left(\frac{1}{3}, -1\right)$ **c.** $(-0.75, 1.5)$

    d. $(3, -2)$ **e.** $\left(-\frac{3}{4}, \frac{1}{2}\right)$

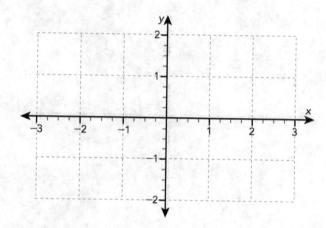

2. Each point in the coordinate plane has an *x*-coordinate and a *y*-coordinate.

    a. Which of the points in Problem 1 have the same *x*-coordinate?

    _____

    b. Do any of the points in Problem 1 have the same *y*-coordinate? If so, which ones?

    _____

Extra Practice continued

3. Look at the ratio of y to x in the points (1.5, −1), $\left(\frac{1}{3}, -1\right)$, (−0.75, 1.5),
(3, −2), and $\left(-\frac{3}{4}, \frac{1}{2}\right)$.

   a. Which of the points have the same ratio $\frac{y}{x}$?

   _____

   b. Give the coordinates of another point with this same ratio.

   _____

   c. Plot the points from part (a) and part (b) on a graph and draw a line
      through them.

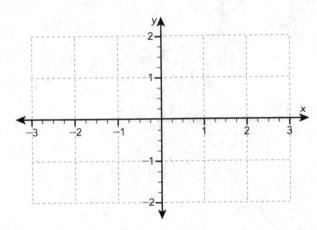

4. Check that the x- and y-coordinates of each of the four points you graphed
in Problem 3 satisfy the formula y = kx for the constant ratio $k = \frac{y}{x}$.

_____

_____

_____

_____

How Steep Is the Line?

Name _____ Class _____ Date _____

Extra Practice

1. Each of the following (x, y) tables is a ratio table. Fill in the missing values and formulas. Identify the constant ratio $\frac{y}{x}$ in each table.

a. Formula: $y = \frac{1}{2}x$

Constant ratio: _____

x	1	2	3	
y	0.5	1		2

b. Formula: _____

Constant ratio: _____

x	1	2		112
y	1		15	112

c. Formula: _____

Constant ratio: $\frac{2}{1} = 2$

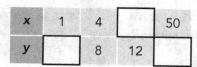

x	1	4		50
y		8	12	

2. Choose one of the formulas and (x, y) tables from Problem 1.

a. Plot at least two points from the table on the coordinate plane.

b. Sketch a straight line that passes through both of the points you plotted.

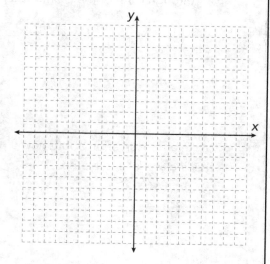

3. What is the coefficient of x in the formula you chose for Problem 2?

_____

_____

Extra Practice continued

4. Each of the following (x, y) tables is a ratio table. Fill in the missing values and formulas. Identify the constant ratio $\frac{y}{x}$ in each table.

a. Formula: _____

Constant ratio: $\frac{3}{1} = 3$

x	y
3	9
13	
16	48
	66

b. Formula: $y = 4x$

Constant ratio: _____

x	y
1	
	36
10	40
	100

c. Formula: _____

Constant ratio: _____

x	y
1	0.25
2	0.5
10	2.5
12	3

5. Choose one of the formulas and (x, y) tables from Problem 4.

a. Plot at least two points from the table on the coordinate plane.

b. Sketch a straight line that passes through both of the points you plotted.

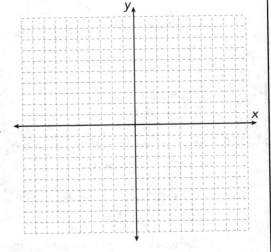

6. Make an observation about how a positive coefficient k and the steepness of the line $y = kx$ are related.

_____

_____

5-4 Introducing Slope

Extra Practice

For formulas of the form $y = kx$, the constant ratio $k = \frac{y}{x}$ is the slope of the line. For example, the slope of the line $y = \frac{2}{3}x$ is $\frac{2}{3}$. You can show these constant ratios by making a graph with a constant slope, or a ratio table for each triangle, using right triangles to show the constant ratio between rise and run.

1. Make a ratio table showing three ordered pairs of x- and y-values that satisfy the formula $y = \frac{2}{3}x$.

2. Sketch three right triangles that represent different ramps with a slope of $\frac{2}{3}$. Use the points in your table for Problem 1 to define the rise and run of each ramp.

3. Sketch a graph on a coordinate plane that represents your three ramps from Problem 2.

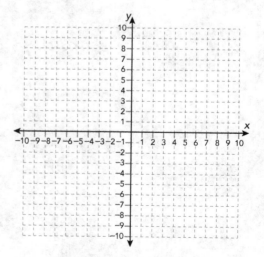

Extra Practice continued

4. Make a ratio table showing three ordered pairs of x- and y-values that satisfy the formula $y = \frac{1}{2}x$.

5. Sketch three right triangles that represent different ramps with a slope of $\frac{1}{2}$. Use the points in your table for Problem 4 to define the rise and run of each ramp.

6. Sketch a graph on the coordinate plane to represent your three ramps from Problem 5.

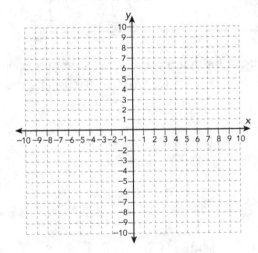

5-5 Graphing Negative Values

Extra Practice

1. Make a table showing at least five ordered pairs of values for a relationship between x and y with each of the following constant ratios.

a. $k = 1$

b. $k = 2$

c. $k = \frac{1}{2}$

d. $k = -1$

e. $k = -2$

f. $k = -\frac{1}{2}$

2. Write a formula to represent each relationship shown in Problem 1.

_____

_____

Extra Practice continued

3. Sketch a graph of the relationship with constant ratio $k = \frac{1}{2}$.

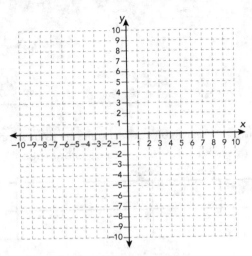

4. On the same coordinate axes you used in Problem 3, sketch a graph of the relationship with constant ratio $k = -2$.

5. Make at least one observation about how the two graphs in Problems 3 and 4 are similar to or different from each other.

_____

_____

_____

_____

5-6 Relationships Without a Constant Ratio

Extra Practice

Consider the following graphs.

GRAPH 1

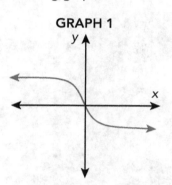

GRAPH 2

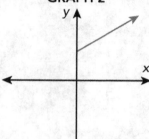

GRAPH 3

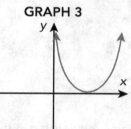

GRAPH 4

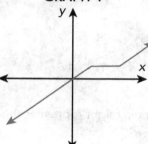

GRAPH 5

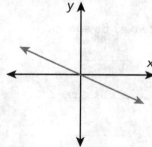

GRAPH 6

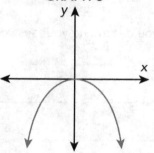

1. Which of the graphs intersect the origin? _____

2. Which one of the graphs represents a proportional relationship? _____

Extra Practice continued

3. Which one of the following tables shows some of the points on the graph of a proportional relationship at the right? The scale is the same on both axes.

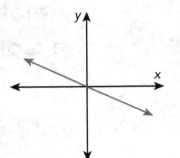

A

x	−10	−2.3	0	1.5	18
y	−40	−9.2	0	6	72

B

x	0	2	5	10	24
y	0	1	3	7	17

C

x	−1.5	−1	0	1.6	3
y	3	2	0	−3.2	−6

D

x	−10.5	−3	0	2.9	12
y	5.25	1.5	0	−1.45	−6

E

x	−8	−2.5	0	3	8
y	4	1.25	0	−2	−6

4. Which formula might represent the proportional relationship in the graph above?

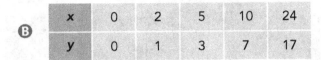

A $y = -2x$ **B** $y = \frac{1}{2}x$ **C** $y = x + \frac{1}{2}$ **D** $y = \frac{1}{2}x$ **E** $y = -\frac{1}{2}x$

5. How did you determine your answer to Problem 4? Be specific.

_____

_____

_____

_____

Name _____ Class _____ Date _____

5-7 Graphs Showing Speed

● Extra Practice

Use this scenario for Problems 1–9: A bicycle rider starts at the top of a hill and rides downhill at a constant speed of 20 miles per hour.

1. Make a table showing five ordered pairs for the time t (in hours) and the distance d (in miles) that the bicycle rider travels when she is riding downhill.

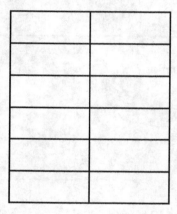

2. Plot the points from your table on the coordinate plane.

3. Does it make sense to connect the points in your graph? If so, draw the line through the points and explain why it makes sense to connect the points. If not, explain why not.

_____

_____

_____

Showing Relationships with Graphs   153   **Extra Practice Lesson 7**

Extra Practice continued

4. Does your graph intersect the origin (0, 0)? Explain.

_____

5. When the value of t doubles, triples, quadruples (is four times as big), and so on, does the value of d also double, triple, quadruple, and so on? Explain.

_____

6. Is the table a ratio table? Explain.

_____

7. Are d and t proportional to each other? Explain.

_____

8. What is the constant of proportionality $\frac{d}{t}$ in this situation?

_____

9. Write a formula to represent the relationship between d and t.

_____

10. If you want to calculate the speed at which you walk to school, what measurements would you take? What units would you use?

_____

_____

11. Label the axes of the graph using the units you chose in the previous problem. What are the units for the speed at which you walk to school?

_____

5-8 Graphing Geometric Relationships

Extra Practice

Use the formulas $P = 4s$ and $s = \frac{1}{4}P$ for Problems 1–3. Both formulas describe the relationship between the following two quantities:

- s, the side of a square
- P, the perimeter of the square

1. What is the constant of proportionality in each formula?

_____

_____

2. Use the graph of $P = 4s$ at the right to approximate these values.

   a. What is P when $s = 2$? _____

   b. What is P when $s = 4$? _____

   c. What is s when $P = 4$? _____

   d. What is s when $P = 12$? _____

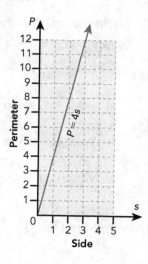

Extra Practice continued

3. Use the graph of $s = \frac{1}{4}P$ at the right to approximate these values.

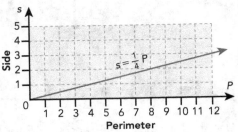

a. What is s when $P = 4$? _____

b. What is s when $P = 12$? _____

c. What is P when $s = 2$? _____

d. What is P when $s = 4$? _____

Use the formulas $C = \pi d$ and $d = \frac{1}{\pi}C$ for Problems 4–5. Both formulas describe the relationship between the following two quantities:

- d, the diameter of a circle
- C, the circumference of the circle

4. What is the constant of proportionality in each formula?

_____

_____

5. Use the graph at the right (which uses 3.14 for π) to approximate these values.

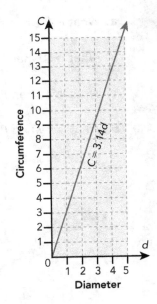

a. What is C when $d = 2$? _____

b. What is C when $d = 4$? _____

c. What is d when $C = 3.14$? _____

d. What is d when $C = 9.42$? _____

Graphing Discrete and Continuous Data

Extra Practice

1. At a local market a farmer sells apples for 30 cents each.

a. Sketch a graph to represent the relationship between the number of apples and the total cost of the apples. Think carefully about whether to connect the points on your graph.

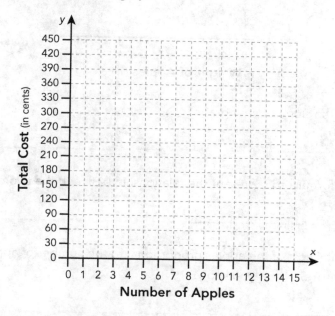

b. What is the slope of a line passing through the points? Say how you know.

_____

c. Write a formula to represent the relationship between the two quantities.

_____

d. Is the total cost of the apples proportional to the number of apples purchased? Say how you know.

_____

_____

Extra Practice continued ——————————————

2. Another farmer is selling apples for $1.50 per pound.

    a. Sketch a graph to represent the relationship between the weight of the apples and the total cost of the apples. Think carefully about whether to connect the points on your graph.

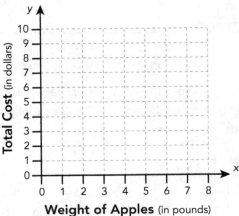

    b. What is the slope of your graph?

    _____

    c. Write a formula to represent the relationship between the two quantities.

    _____

    d. Is the total cost of the apples proportional to the number of apples purchased? Say how you know.

    _____

3. Does the situation in Problem 2 involve discrete or continuous data? Does it involve a constant decrease or a constant increase? Explain your answers.

_____

_____

_____

5-10 Progress Check

Extra Practice

If you need help with the following problems, sketch a diagram, make an (x, y) table, or write a formula to represent the relationship between quantities.

1. A plant that starts out 0 inches tall grows 0.5 inches per week. After x weeks, the plant is y inches tall.

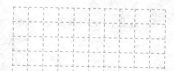

   a. Sketch a graph that represents the relationship between x and y. Think carefully about whether the graph should be discrete or continuous, and label the axes with the quantities in the relationship.

   b. Tell whether the relationship is proportional and explain your answer.

_____

_____

2. An office supply store is having a sale, and erasers are on sale for $0.25 each. The total cost of x erasers is y dollars.

   a. Sketch a graph that represents the relationship between x and y. Think carefully about whether the graph should be discrete or continuous, and label the axes with the quantities in the relationship.

   b. Tell whether the relationship is proportional and explain your answer.

_____

_____

Extra Practice continued

3. Chen's younger brother, Winston, is 12 years old and 57 inches tall. Chen is 15 years old and 68 inches tall. His older sister, Amy, is 17 years old and 65 inches tall. His older brother, Jong, is 19 years old and 67 inches tall. A person who is x years old has a height of y inches.

   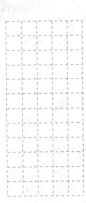

   a. Sketch a graph that represents the relationship between x and y. Think carefully about whether the graph should be discrete or continuous, and label the axes with the quantities in the relationship.

   b. Tell whether the relationship is proportional and explain your answer.

   _____

   _____

4. A bicycle rider travels at a constant speed of 12 miles per hour. After x hours, he has traveled y miles.

   a. Sketch a graph that represents the relationship between x and y. Think carefully about whether the graph should be discrete or continuous, and label the axes with the quantities in the relationship.

   b. Tell whether the relationship is proportional and explain your answer.

   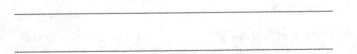

   _____

   _____

Extra Practice

For Problems 1–6, match the described situation or relationship to one or more of the tables below. Write the letter of the table next to the description.

A

x	0	1	2	3	4	5
y	8	7.2	6.4	5.6	4.8	4

B

x	0	1	2	3	4	5
y	3	11	19	27	35	43

C

x	0	1	2	3	4	5
y	0	8	16	24	32	40

1. A tank contains 3 gallons of water. You add water to the tank at a constant rate of 8 gallons per minute. _____

2. You add water to an empty tank at a constant rate of 8 gallons every minute. _____

3. A water tank contains 8 gallons of water. You pour water out of the tank at a rate of 0.8 gallon per minute. _____

4. Which of the tables indicates a proportional relationship? _____

5. Which of the tables indicates a linear relationship? _____

6. Which of the tables indicates a relationship with a constant decrease? _____

Extra Practice continued

7. a. Sketch a graph to represent each of the water tank situations. (The tables are repeated below.)

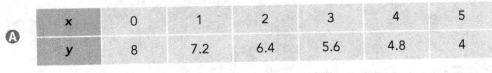

A

x	0	1	2	3	4	5
y	8	7.2	6.4	5.6	4.8	4

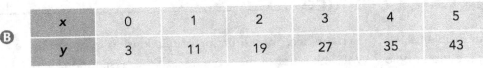

B

x	0	1	2	3	4	5
y	3	11	19	27	35	43

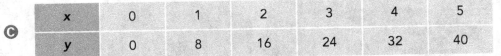

C

x	0	1	2	3	4	5
y	0	8	16	24	32	40

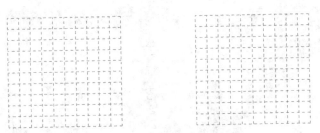 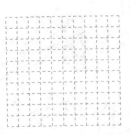

b. Are your graphs discrete or continuous? Say why.

_____

_____

c. What is the slope (constant increase or decrease) of each of your graphs?

_____

d. What is the y-intercept of each of your graphs?

_____

e. Do your graphs show a constant decrease or increase?

_____

_____

Name _____ Class _____ Date _____

5-12 Focus on Slope

Extra Practice

1. What is *m*, the coefficient of *x*, in each of these equations?

$y = \frac{1}{2}x - 1$ $\qquad\qquad$ $y = -2x - 1$

_____

2. Identify two points on the line $y = \frac{1}{2}x - 1$ by finding two pairs of *x*- and *y*-values that satisfy the equation. Confirm that $m = \frac{\text{change in } y}{\text{change in } x}$ for the *x*- and *y*-coordinates of the points.

_____

3. Identify two points on the line $y = -2x - 1$ by finding two pairs of *x*- and *y*-values that satisfy the equation. Confirm that $m = \frac{\text{change in } y}{\text{change in } x}$ for the *x*- and *y*-coordinates of the points.

_____

_____

4. Look at the two lines at right. Confirm that the four points you identified in Problems 2 and 3 are, in fact, on the lines. Then write one observation about the lines.

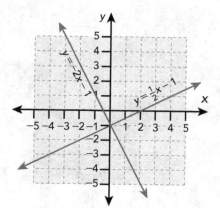

_____

_____

Extra Practice continued

You know that the slope of a line defined by a slope-intercept equation of the form $y = mx + b$ is m, the coefficient of x.

You also know that in the equation $y = mx + b$, the y-intercept of the line is b.

In proportional relationships, b is 0 and m is equal to the constant of proportionality, $\frac{y}{x}$.

5. Write a slope-intercept equation and sketch a graph of a proportional relationship with a constant of proportionality of −1.

_____

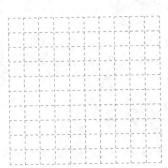

6. Write a slope-intercept equation and sketch a graph of a linear relationship with a slope of −1 and a y-intercept of −1.

_____

5-13 Parallel and Perpendicular Lines

Extra Practice

1. **a.** Write a slope-intercept equation of a proportional relationship with a constant of proportionality of $\frac{2}{5}$.

   _____

   b. Sketch the graph.

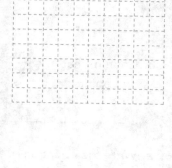

2. **a.** Write a slope-intercept equation of a linear relationship with a slope of -2.5 and a y-intercept of -3.

   _____

   b. Sketch the graph.

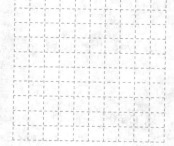

3. Look at the graphs you sketched in Problems 1 and 2. These lines *look* perpendicular. Say how you can be *sure* that they are perpendicular.

   _____

   _____

Extra Practice continued

4. a. Identify two points on the line $y = \frac{2}{5}x$ by finding two pairs of x- and y-values that satisfy the equation.

_____

b. Confirm that $m = \frac{\text{change in } y}{\text{change in } x}$ for the x- and y-coordinates of your two points.

_____

5. a. Identify two points on the line $y = -2.5x - 3$ by finding two pairs of x- and y-values that satisfy the equation.

_____

b. Confirm that $m = \frac{\text{change in } y}{\text{change in } x}$ for the x- and y-coordinates of your two points.

_____

6. a. Write the equation of a line parallel to $y = \frac{2}{5}x$.

_____

b. Write the equation of a line perpendicular to $y = -2.5x - 3$.

_____

c. Do the equations you wrote for part (a) and part (b) represent parallel or perpendicular lines? Explain your answer.

_____

_____

5-14 The Water Tank Problem

Extra Practice

1. Complete the table for a tank that fills up at a rate of 240 liters per minute.

Pumping Time (minutes)	t	0	10	20	30	40	50
Volume of Water (liters)	V	0					

2. The height in meters *h* of the water tank is related to the volume in liters *V* by the equation $V = 3000h$.

   a. What information is provided by this equation?

   _____

   _____

   b. Add a third row to the table from Problem 1 and fill in the corresponding values for the heights of the water in the tank after *t* minutes of pumping.

3. Use your table to estimate how long it would take to fill up an empty tank to a height of 2 meters.

   _____

4. Use your table to estimate the volume of the water when the height of the water is 3.6 m.

   _____

Extra Practice continued

5. Complete the following table for a different tank that fills up at a rate of 150 liters per minute.

Pumping Time (minutes) t	0	10	20	30	40	50
Volume of Water (liters) V	0					

6. The height in centimeters *h* of the water tank is related to the volume *V* by the equation $V = 50h$.

  a. What information is provided by this equation?

  _____

  _____

  b. Add a third row to the table from Problem 5 and fill in the corresponding values for the heights of the water in the tank after *t* minutes of pumping.

7. Use your table to estimate how long it would take to fill up an empty tank to a height of 3 meters.

  _____

8. Use your table to estimate the volume when the height of the water is 10 cm.

  _____

5-15 The Algebra of the Water Tank Problem

Extra Practice

1. The equation $V = 400t$ represents the relationship between the volume of water V filling a tank at time t. Volume is measured in liters and time is measured in minutes.

   a. How much water is in the tank at the start?

   _____

   b. At what rate is the volume of water in the truck's tank changing?

   _____

   c. If the tank has a capacity of 9600 liters, how long will it take to fill the tank?

   _____

   d. How long will it take to fill one-third of the tank?

   _____

2. The equation $V = 400t + 4000$ represents the relationship between the volume of water V in a second tank at time t. Volume is measured in liters and time is measured in minutes.

   a. How much water is in the tank at the start?

   _____

   b. At what rate is the volume of water in the truck's tank changing?

   _____

   c. If the tank has a capacity of 9600 liters, how long will it take to fill the tank?

   _____

   d. How long will it take to fill one-half of the tank?

   _____

Extra Practice continued

3. The equation $y = 20{,}000 - 400x$ represents the relationship between the volume of water y in the truck's tank at time x. Volume is measured in liters and time is measured in minutes.

   a. How much water is in the truck at the start?

   _____

   b. At what rate is the volume of water in the truck's tank changing?

   _____

   c. How long will it take to empty the tank?

   _____

   d. How long will it take for the volume of water in the truck to drop to 1600 liters?

   _____

   e. How much water is left in the truck after 20 minutes?

   _____

5-16 Solving Systems by Graphing

Extra Practice

Use the following situation for Problems 1–4.

Lydia is deciding how she will commute to work. She can drive and buy a monthly pass at a parking garage for $195, while paying $4 a day in tolls during her drive. She can also take the light rail for $10.50 a day.

1. Let x be the number of days Lydia commutes to work in a month. Let y be the total cost of her commute. Write an equation to represent each of her choices.

   _____

2. Graph the equations from Problem 1. Estimate the point of intersection. What does this point represent?

   _____

   _____

3. How do you think Lydia should commute to work? Use the graph to support your answer.

   _____

   _____

4. How can you check to see if your estimate from Problem 2 is the actual point of intersection of the two graphs?

   _____

   _____

5. If Lydia commutes 30 days in one month, what is the cost of commuting?

   _____

Extra Practice continued

Use the following situation for Problems 6–10.

Roberto is saving money to buy a certain antique car. The price of the car is $4300, but the price decreases by $100 every month. Roberto currently has $700 in his savings account. He is able to save $300 every month. How long before Roberto has enough money to buy the car?

6. What are the two quantities that vary in this situation?

_____

7. Assign a variable to each quantity in Problem 6. Then write a system of equations to model the situation.

_____

_____

8. Graph the equations from Problem 7. Estimate the point of intersection.

_____

9. Substitute the x-value of your intersection point into the equations you wrote for Problem 7. How close was your estimate of the y-value?

_____

_____

_____

10. Explain how the point of intersection represents the answer to the question that is posed in the scenario.

_____

_____

_____

_____

5-17 Interpreting Graphs

Extra Practice

1. These two graphs show the height of a growing plant. Graph 1 uses line segments to join points. Graph 2 uses a single, smooth curve.

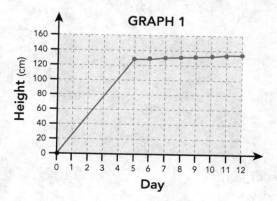

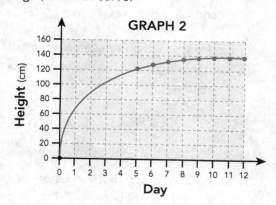

a. Use Graph 1 to estimate the height of the plant on day 3. _____

b. Use Graph 2 to estimate the height of the plant on day 3. _____

c. Use Graph 1 to estimate the age of the plant when it reached a height of 60 cm. _____

d. Use Graph 2 to estimate the age of the plant when it reached a height of 60 cm. _____

e. Which graph do you think gives a better approximation of the plant's growth? Why?

_____

_____

Showing Relationships with Graphs 173 **Extra Practice Lesson 17**

Name _____ Class _____ Date _____

Extra Practice continued _____

This table shows the total cost per month of leaving lights on for different numbers of hours per day. Use this table for Problems 2–4.

Hours per Day	5	7	9
Cost per Month	$5.10	$7.14	$9.18

2. **a.** Sketch a graph that estimates the cost of leaving the lights on for 3.5 hours per day. Choose an appropriate scale and label the axes.

   b. Use your graph to estimate the cost of leaving the lights on for 3.5 hours per day.

   _____

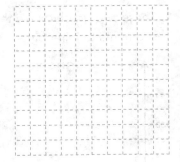

3. **a.** Sketch a graph that estimates the cost of leaving the lights on for 20 hours per day. Choose an appropriate scale and label the axes.

   b. Use your graph to estimate the cost of leaving the lights on for 20 hours per day.

   _____

4. Is either of your graphs linear? Is either of your graphs proportional? If so, which one(s)?

_____

Name _____ Class _____ Date _____

5-18 The Unit in Review

Extra Practice

1. Look at the (x, y) table below.

x	−10	−4	−1	1	4	10
y	−4.6	−0.4	1.7	3.1	5.2	9.4

a. Write the slope-intercept equation for the line that passes through the points in the table by finding the slope between any two points and then finding the y-intercept.

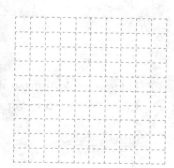

_____

b. Sketch a graph of the points in the table and draw a line through them. How does the line compare to the equation you wrote in part (a)?

_____

_____

2. Consider the graphs of the nine equations listed below.

Ⓐ $y = -2x + 6$ Ⓑ $y = 0.5x + 3$ Ⓒ $y = -0.5x - 3$

Ⓓ $y = -\frac{1}{5}x + 3$ Ⓔ $y = -\frac{1}{2}x + 4$ Ⓕ $y = \frac{1}{2}x - 1$

Ⓖ $y = 3x - 0.5$ Ⓗ $y = -0.5x + 5$ Ⓘ $y = 2x + 3$

a. Which of the graphs are parallel to the line $y = -0.5x + 3$? _____

b. Which of the graphs are perpendicular to the line $y = -0.5x + 3$?

_____

3. Andrew is deciding whether he should purchase a membership to a museum. Admission to the museum is $15 for nonmembers and $10 for members. The membership fee is $60.

a. Write a system of equations to model the situation.

_____

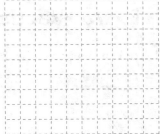

b. Graph the equations from part (a). Estimate the point of intersection. What does this point represent?

_____

_____

_____

c. Do you think Andrew should buy the museum membership? Use the graph to support your answer.

_____

_____

4. On the left grid, sketch a graph that shows a proportional relationship. On the right grid, sketch a graph that shows a line with a negative slope. Write the equation for each graph.

_____ _____

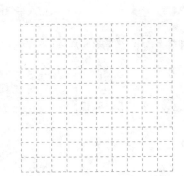 

6-1 Representing Quantities with Expressions

■ Extra Practice

In Problems 1–5, sketch a diagram to represent the description. Label your diagrams with the numbers and variables in the description.

1. There are n booklets in a stack. Each booklet is 12 mm thick.

2. There are 12 booklets in a stack. Each booklet is x mm thick.

3. There are 5 more girls than boys in the class. There are b boys in the class.

4. There are 5 fewer boys than girls in the class. There are g girls in the class.

5. There are 5 boys in the class. There are m more girls than boys in the class.

Extra Practice continued

Write variable expressions that represent the quantities identified below.

6. There are *n* booklets in a stack. Each booklet is 12 mm thick. What is the height, in millimeters, of the stack of booklets?

_____

7. There are 12 booklets in a stack. Each booklet is *x* mm thick. What is the height, in millimeters, of the stack of booklets?

_____

8. There are 5 more girls than boys in the class. There are *b* boys in the class. What is the total number of students in the class?

_____

9. There are 5 fewer boys than girls in the class. There are *g* girls in the class. What is the total number of students in the class?

_____

10. There are 5 boys in the class. There are *m* more girls than boys in the class. What is the total number of students in the class?

_____

11. Dwayne has *d* dollars in a bank account. He deposits $150 and then pays a bill online for $29.99. What is the amount left in his bank account?

_____

12. Keesha has *d* dollars in a bank account. She pays a bill online for $45. Then she deposits $35.00. What is the amount left in her bank account?

_____

13. In Problem 12, what positive integer values for *d* indicate that Keesha has overdrawn her bank account?

_____

6-2 Evaluating Expressions

Extra Practice

1. A shelf contains a row of x DVDs in cases that are each 9 millimeters thick and y boxed sets that are each 27 millimeters thick.

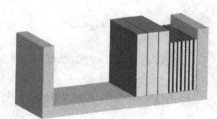

 a. Write an expression for the width, in millimeters, of x DVDs in cases and y boxed sets.

    _____

 b. What are the terms of the expression?

    _____

 c. What do the terms represent in the situation?

    _____

    _____

 d. What are the coefficients of the terms?

    _____

 e. What do the coefficients represent in the situation?

    _____

    _____

 f. If the shelf is 0.5 meters in length, how many boxed sets will fit on the shelf? How many DVD cases?

    _____

Extra Practice continued

2. A shelf contains a row of x paperback books that are each 16 millimeters thick.

   a. Write an expression for the width, in millimeters, of x paperback books. _____

   b. What are the terms of the expression? _____

   c. What do the terms represent in the situation?

   _____

   d. What is the coefficient of the term? _____

   e. What does the coefficient represent in the situation?

   _____

   _____

3. Suppose Dwayne wants to buy x regular pencils for 20 cents each and y mechanical pencils for 85 cents each.

   a. Write a variable expression using x and y for the total cost of x regular pencils and y mechanical pencils.

   _____

   b. What do the coefficients in the variable expression represent?

   _____

   _____

   c. What is the total cost for 5 regular pencils and 1 mechanical pencil?

   _____

   d. What is the total cost for 2 regular pencils and 3 mechanical pencils?

   _____

   e. How many regular pencils can he buy for $3.40? How many mechanical pencils can be bought for the same amount?

   _____

6-3 Exponents

Extra Practice

1. Complete the table.

Expression	Base	Exponent	Value
6^3			
	0.2	2	
		3	27
	−8		4096

2. How many factors of 7 are in each of these expressions?

a. $7 \cdot 7 \cdot 7 \cdot 7 \cdot 7 \cdot 7 \cdot 7 \cdot 7$

b. 7^4

_____

_____

c. $(7^6)^2$

d. 7^x

_____

_____

e. $-(7)^3$

f. $7x^2$

_____

_____

g. $(-7x^3)^3$

h. $(7^2 x^4)^4$

_____

_____

i. $(7^x y^2)^2$

_____

3. Explain how you can evaluate $(\sqrt{12{,}345})^2$ without using a calculator.

_____

_____

Extra Practice continued

4. Decide if each of the following is true or false. Write a brief justification for each choice.

   a. In the expression 58^2, the exponent is 58.

   _____

   b. $15^3 = 45$

   _____

   c. $72 = 2^3 \cdot 3^2$

   _____

   d. The expression 2^x is equivalent to $x \cdot x$.

   _____

   _____

   e. $(-8)^2 = 8^2$

   _____

   f. $(-6)^3 = 6^3$

   _____

   _____

   g. $3^4 = -3^4$

   _____

Operations with Exponents

Extra Practice

1. Complete this table.

Exponent Form	Expanded Form
$2x^5$	
	$5 \cdot y \cdot y \cdot p$
	$10 \cdot d \cdot p \cdot p$
$7x^5y^2$	
$(7x^3)(8y)^2$	
$(-4)^2m^3$	

2. Evaluate each of these expressions using the values $a = -2$ and $b = 3$.

  a. $2a^5$ **b.** ab^2 **c.** a^b **d.** $(-ab)^2$

_____   _____   _____   _____

3. Simplify these expressions by adding or subtracting exponents.

  a. $x^4 \cdot x^3$ **b.** $m^8 \div m^6$ **c.** $\dfrac{n^5p^2}{n}$ **d.** $\dfrac{k^7b^8}{b^5} \cdot \dfrac{k^2}{b}$

_____   _____   _____   _____

  e. $\dfrac{y^6y^4}{y^9}$ **f.** $p^2 \cdot p^3 \cdot p^0$ **g.** $\dfrac{g^{12}}{g^7} \cdot \dfrac{g^8}{g}$ **h.** $\dfrac{h}{k^4} \cdot \dfrac{k^6}{hk}$

_____   _____   _____   _____

Extra Practice continued

4. Decide if each of the following is true or false. Write a brief justification for each choice.

a. $n^7 \cdot n^2 = n^{14}$

_____

_____

b. $64^0 = 64$

_____

c. $9^m \div 9^n = 9^{m-n}$

_____

_____

d. $2^3 \cdot a^7 = 8a^7$

_____

e. $0^0 = 1$

_____

f. $\frac{x^6}{x^2} = x^3$

_____

g. $ab^3 \cdot a^4 b^3 = a^7 b^6$

_____

_____

6-5 Expressions and Area Models

Extra Practice

1. a. Calculate $2^2 + 5^2$. _____

    b. Sketch a geometric figure with an area that can be represented by $2^2 + 5^2$.

2. a. Calculate $(2 + 5)^2$. _____

    b. Sketch a geometric figure with an area that can be represented by $(2 + 5)^2$.

Extra Practice continued

3. **a.** Calculate $(3 \cdot 2) + 7$. _____

   b. Sketch a geometric figure with an area that can be represented
   by $(3 \cdot 2) + 7$.

4. **a.** Calculate $3(2 + 7)$. _____

   b. Sketch a geometric figure with an area that can be represented
   by $3(2 + 7)$.

5. Evaluate these expressions for $d = -3$.

   a. d^2 **b.** $-d^2$ **c.** $(-d)^2$

   _____   _____   _____

   d. $-3d$ **e.** $(-2d)^2$ **f.** $-2d^2$

   _____   _____   _____

6-6 Combining Like Terms

 Extra Practice

In Problems 1–14, write the additive inverse of each expression.

1. x

_____

2. $-x$

_____

3. $-(-x)$

_____

4. $10x^4$

_____

5. $-10x^4$

_____

6. $-(-10x^4)$

_____

7. $8y^4$

_____

8. $-5z^5$

_____

9. $-3y^2$

_____

10. $-(-3y^2)$

_____

11. $2m$

_____

12. $-2m$

_____

13. $-(6y)$

_____

14. $-6y$

_____

Extra Practice continued

In Problems 15–18, use the Distributive Property and the Commutative Property of Multiplication to rewrite each of the expressions.

15. $9y - 8y$

_____

Samples

$4a + 8a = a(4 + 8) = (4 + 8)a$

$2m - m = m(2 + -1) = (2 + -1)m$

$x^4 - 10x^4 = x^4(1 + -10) = (1 + -10)x^4$

16. $z - 5z$

_____

17. $9y^4 - 8y^4$

_____

18. $z^5 - 5z^5$

_____

19. Simplify these expressions by combining like terms. Use the Distributive Property and the Commutative Property, as you did in Problems 15–18, but simplify as far as possible.

a. $7x + 2x$ **b.** $7x^2 - 2x^2$ **c.** $7x + (-2x)$

_____   _____   _____

d. $7x^2 - (-2x^2)$ **e.** $-7x - 2x$ **f.** $-7x^2 + (-2x^2)$

_____   _____   _____

g. $-7x^2 + 2x^2$ **h.** $-7x - (-2x)$

_____   _____

6-7 Combining Quantities

Extra Practice

1. State whether the inequalities are *true* or *false*. For each inequality that is false, rewrite it so that it is true using one of these methods:

- Switch the inequality symbol.
- Change the quantity with larger units.
- Change the quantity with smaller units.

Use each of the methods listed above in at least one of these inequalities.

a. 5 yd < 17 ft

_____

b. $13.22 < 1299 cents

_____

c. 28 ounces > 4 cups

_____

d. 72 m > 7199 cm

_____

e. 3.5 hr < 220 min

_____

f. 72 km < 7201 m

_____

g. 3323 cm < 32 m

_____

Extra Practice continued

The inequalities in Problems 2 and 3 are written with variable expressions on either side of the inequality sign. Evaluate the expressions for the given values and state whether the inequalities are true or false for those values.

2. $6a < 12b$

    a. $a = 10$, $b = 5$ **b.** $a = 100$, $b = 51$ **c.** $a = 9$, $b = 4$

    _____   _____   _____

3. $2x + 1 > x^2$

    a. $x = 1$ **b.** $x = 2$ **c.** $x = 3$

    _____   _____   _____

4. Rosa is buying walnuts and pecans for a granola recipe. Walnuts cost $2.65 per pound and pecans cost $0.18 per ounce. There are 16 ounces in 1 pound.

    a. Write an expression for the total cost of x pounds of walnuts and y ounces of pecans.

    _____

    b. What is the total cost of 2 pounds of walnuts and 24 ounces of pecans?

    _____

    c. If Rosa buys 2 pounds of walnuts and 24 ounces of pecans, what is the total weight of the walnuts and pecans? First write your answer in pounds, then write your answer in ounces.

    _____

    d. Which type of nut is more expensive, walnuts or pecans? What is the difference in their cost per pound?

    _____

6-8 Adding and Subtracting Expressions

Extra Practice

1. Use the Distributive Property to simplify these expressions.

   a. $-5(x - y)$ **b.** $-5(x - 3)$ **c.** $-5(20 - 3)$

   _____   _____   _____

2. Student work is shown below.

   $(4x + 7) - (3x - 2)$

          $= 4x + 7 - 3x - 2$

          $= 4x - 3x + 7 - 2$

          $= (4 - 3)x + 5$

          $= x + 5$

   a. Circle the first line of the solution in which the student made a mistake.

   b. Explain the misconception that led to the mistake.

   _____

   _____

   c. Write the correct solution.

   _____

   _____

   _____

   d. What advice would you give to this student?

   _____

   _____

   _____

Extra Practice continued

3. Student work is shown below.

$(3 - 2n) - 2(7n - 5)$

$= 3 - 2n + -2 \cdot 7n - -2 \cdot -5$

$= 3 - 2n + -14n + -10$

$= 3 + -10 - 2n + -14n$

$= (-2 + -14)n + 3 - 10$

$= -16n - 7$

a. Circle the first line of the solution in which the student made a mistake.

b. What was the mistake?

_____

_____

c. Write the correct solution.

_____

_____

_____

_____

_____

_____

4. Circle the expressions below that are equal.

$2 - (n - 3)$ $2 + (-n) - 3$ $2 - n + 3$ $n - 5$

$-2n - 6$ $2 - (-3 + n)$ $-2n + 6$ $5 - n$

6-9 Parentheses and Exponents

Extra Practice

1. Decide whether each equation is true or false and then write an explanation to justify your choice.

a. $(ab)^2 = ab^2$

_____

b. $(a + b)^2 = a^2 + b^2$

_____

_____

c. $\left(\dfrac{a}{b}\right)^2 = \dfrac{(a)^2}{b}$

_____

d. $(-a)^2 = a^2$

_____

e. $(-a)^3 = a^3$

_____

f. $\left(\sqrt{a}\right)^2 = a$

_____

_____

g. $(ab)^0 = 1$

_____

h. $a(b)^0 = 1$

_____

Extra Practice continued

2. Evaluate these expressions without using a calculator.

    a. $(-3)^4$ **b.** $-(3)^4$

    _____   _____

3. Write the simplest possible exponential expression for the area of the triangle with perpendicular height $3(xy)^5z$ and base $8\left(\dfrac{xy^2}{z}\right)^3$.

    _____

4. Write each expression in exponential form. Do not use parentheses in parts (a)–(c).

    a. $(5^3)^7$ **b.** $(4m^0)^2$

    _____   _____

    c. $\left(\dfrac{3^6}{5^3}\right)^2$ **d.** $[(-6)^5]^3$

    _____   _____

5. Write each expression in exponential form, without parentheses.

    a. $(x^2yz^4)^5$ **b.** $(mn^6)^3m^4$

    _____   _____

    c. $(a^2b^3)(ab^2)^2$ **d.** $\left(\dfrac{x^3y^4}{xy^3}\right)^3$

    _____   _____

6. In Problem 5(d), is it easier to simplify the terms in parentheses before applying the exponent? Say why.

    _____

    _____

    _____

    _____

6-10 Negative Exponents

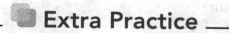 Extra Practice

1. Use the properties of negative exponents to write each number as a fraction with two integers.

   a. 4^{-3}

   _____

   b. $(-2)^{-4}$

   _____

   c. $2^{-1} + 4^{-2}$

   _____

   d. $\frac{5^{-2}}{3^{-1}}$

   _____

   e. $(0.25 + 2.75)^{-2}$

   _____

   f. $(2^{-3} \cdot 4^2)(2^{-2} \cdot 4^{-5})$

   _____

2. Which of these expressions are equal to $\frac{1}{3}$? Circle the correct answer(s).

   a. 1^{-3}

   b. 3^{-1}

   c. $(-3)^1$

3. Which of these expressions are equal to 2^{-1}? Circle the correct answer(s).

   a. $-\frac{1}{2}$

   b. $\frac{1}{2}$

   c. $(-2)^1$

4. Which of these expressions are equal to $\frac{3^2}{3^{-3}}$? Circle the correct answer(s).

   a. 3^5

   b. 3^{-1}

   c. 3^1

Extra Practice continued _____

5. Write each of these expressions using positive exponents.

a. 8^{-2}

_____

b. p^{-1}

_____

c. $2(m)^{-4}$

_____

d. $(2m)^{-4}$

_____

e. $\dfrac{1}{x^{-3}}$

_____

f. $\dfrac{j^{-7}}{k^6}$

_____

6. Write each of these expressions using negative exponents.

a. $\dfrac{1}{7^3}$

_____

b. 5^2

_____

c. $\dfrac{0.6}{P}$

_____

d. $(-4)^5$

_____

e. $\dfrac{m^5}{n^4}$

_____

f. $\dfrac{-1}{h^8}$

_____

g. $\dfrac{1}{6^4}$

_____

h. 4^3

_____

6-11 Scientific Notation

Extra Practice

1. Write these numbers in scientific notation.

    a. 420,000

    _____

    b. −1270

    _____

    c. 0.0000032

    _____

    d. 0.00162

    _____

    e. −16,200,000

    _____

    f. −0.00000000012

    _____

    g. −3.95

    _____

    h. 893,000,000,000,000

    _____

2. Use a *greater than* or *less than* symbol to complete the following statements.

    a. $1.0075 \cdot 10^{11}$ _____ 98,000,000,000

    b. $4.5 \cdot 10^{8}$ _____ 460,000,000

    c. 0.00000246 _____ $2.46 \cdot 10^{-7}$

    d. $-1.002 \cdot 10^{7}$ _____ $-9.998 \cdot 10^{6}$

    e. 0.0000599 _____ $5.99 \cdot 10^{-6}$

    f. $-6.78 \cdot 10^{-5}$ _____ −0.0000876

Extra Practice continued _____

3. Convert these numbers from scientific notation to standard form.

a. $7.05 \cdot 10^2$

b. $4.685 \cdot 10^{-1}$

c. $1.75 \cdot 10^{10}$

_____

_____

_____

d. $7.05 \cdot 10^{-2}$

e. $4.4275 \cdot 10^8$

f. $2.0 \cdot 10^{-9}$

_____

_____

_____

4. Rewrite the multiplication or division problem in scientific notation. Then use the Associative Property of Multiplication to find the product. Express the product in standard notation. Do not use a calculator.

a. $1600 \cdot 0.00025$

_____

_____

b. $8{,}000{,}000{,}000 \cdot 0.00000034$

_____

_____

c. $0.0000072 \div 0.0000000006$

_____

_____

d. $25{,}600{,}000 \div 800{,}000{,}000$

_____

_____

e. $0.0002 \cdot 202{,}000$

_____

_____

f. $0.202 \div 0.0002$

_____

_____

6-12 Estimating Square Roots

Extra Practice

1. Calculate a value for x that makes each equation true.

    a. $x^2 = 9$ **b.** $x^2 = 64$

    _____   _____

    c. $x^2 = 0.81$ **d.** $x^2 = 0.0025$

    _____   _____

2. This square has an area of 45 square meters and a side length of x.

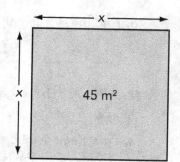

    a. What is the smallest perfect square that is greater than 45 and the largest perfect square that is less than 45?

    _____

    b. Use your answer from part (a) to determine which two whole numbers the value of x must lie between.

    _____

    c. Find the side length accurate to one decimal place.

    _____

    d. Find the side length accurate to two decimal places.

    _____

Extra Practice continued

3. This square has an area of 72 square meters and a side length of *x*.

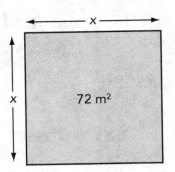

a. What is the smallest perfect square that is greater than 72 and the largest perfect square that is less than 72?

_____

b. Use your answer from part (a) to determine which two whole numbers the value of *x* must lie between.

_____

c. Find the side length accurate to one decimal place.

_____

d. Find the side length accurate to two decimal places.

_____

4. Ms. Reynolds challenged her students to calculate the dimensions of the cube below.

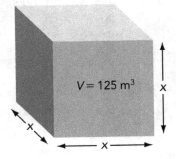

a. Dwayne remembered that the formula for the volume of a cube is $V = x^3$ or $V = x \cdot x \cdot x$. Find the side length of the cube.

_____

b. If the volume of a cube is 64 m³, what is the length of a side?

_____

c. If the volume of a cube is 216 m³, what is the length of a side?

_____

6-13 The Pythagorean Theorem

Extra Practice

1. Use the squares lettered from A to O to form three sets of related diagrams and statements. Each set will have:

- A diagram of a right triangle
- A statement about the right angle
- A statement about the hypotenuse
- A calculation to determine the length of segment *AC*
- A calculation to determine the length of segment *AB*

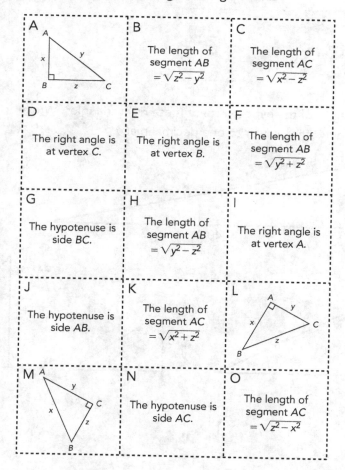

A	**B** The length of segment AB $= \sqrt{z^2 - y^2}$	**C** The length of segment AC $= \sqrt{x^2 - z^2}$
D The right angle is at vertex *C*.	**E** The right angle is at vertex *B*.	**F** The length of segment AB $= \sqrt{y^2 + z^2}$
G The hypotenuse is side *BC*.	**H** The length of segment AB $= \sqrt{y^2 - z^2}$	**I** The right angle is at vertex *A*.
J The hypotenuse is side *AB*.	**K** The length of segment AC $= \sqrt{x^2 + z^2}$	**L**
M	**N** The hypotenuse is side *AC*.	**O** The length of segment AC $= \sqrt{z^2 - x^2}$

Set 1: _____   Set 2: _____   Set 3: _____

Extra Practice continued

2. Use a calculator to help you check whether these sets of integers satisfy the Pythagorean Theorem. For any that do, sketch and label a corresponding right triangle.

a. {12, 16, 20}

_____

b. {4, 5, 6}

_____

c. {8, 15, 17}

_____

d. {7, 23, 24}

_____

e. {16, 20, 25}

_____

3. Label the length of the hypotenuse of these right triangles. Where necessary, round the answer to one decimal place.

a.

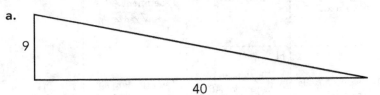

9

40

b.

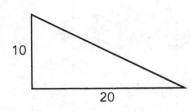

10

20

c.

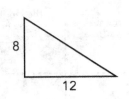

8

12

d.

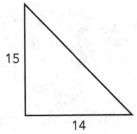

15

14

6-14 Applying the Pythagorean Theorem

🔲 Extra Practice

Consider each statement below and decide if it is true or false. Provide an explanation for your choice using diagrams, algebra, and words.

1. The two legs of a right triangle measure 7 in. and 8 in. respectively. The hypotenuse measures 15 in.

_____

_____

_____

2. The hypotenuse of a right triangle measures 15 in. and one of the legs of the triangle measures 12 in. The length of the third side cannot be calculated.

_____

_____

_____

3. The width of a rectangular gate is 5 m and its height is 1.5 m. The longest diagonal across the gate measures 5.22 m.

_____

_____

_____

Extra Practice continued

4. The length of the slant height of a cone is known, as well as the diameter of the base of the cone. The perpendicular height of the cone can be calculated using this information.

_____

_____

_____

_____

_____

_____

5. If three numbers a, b, and c (where $a < b < c$) fit the Pythagorean Theorem $c^2 = a^2 + b^2$ then they represent the side lengths of a right triangle.

_____

_____

6. If three numbers a, b, and c (where $c > a$ and $c > b$) fit the inequality $c^2 < a^2 + b^2$ then they represent the side lengths of an obtuse triangle.

_____

_____

7. If three numbers a, b, and c (where $a < b < c$) fit the Pythagorean Theorem $c^2 = a^2 + b^2$ then the three numbers $2a$, $2b$, and $2c$ also fit the Pythagoream Theorem.

_____

_____

_____

_____

6-15 Progress Check

Extra Practice

1. For each situation, write an expression that represents the quantity described. Use conventions to write your expressions correctly.

a. Each pea pod contains 3 peas.
Quantity: The number of peas in p pea pods

_____

b. Rosa is scheduled to work 15 hours in a given week at a hardware store.
Quantity: The number of hours Rosa works if she works t hours of overtime

_____

c. Every ride on the camel requires 4 tickets. Dwayne has 20 tickets.
Quantity: The number of tickets Dwayne has after c camel rides

_____

2. Write two equivalent expressions for the quantity represented by this area model. State which number property or properties tell you your expressions are equivalent.

x	x	x	x	6	6

x 10

_____

_____

_____

_____

3. Simplify the expression $10(x + 4y) - 5(y - 3x)$. Use the Commutative Property of Addition and the Distributive Property to combine like terms.

_____

_____

_____

Extra Practice continued

4. Write these numbers in scientific notation.

    a. 0.0000061

    b. −5,798,200,000

_____   _____

5. Lisa is making a picture frame using thin wooden strips of different thicknesses. Some of the wood strips are cut to 12 millimeters thick and the other strips are cut to 3 centimeters thick.

    a. If she uses 8 of the 12-mm strips and 4 of the 3-cm strips, what is the total width of the picture frame in millimeters? _____

    b. Write a variable expression for the total width in millimeters of the picture frame if she uses x of the 12-mm strips and y of the 3-cm strips. _____

    c. Check your answer to part (a) by evaluating your expression in part (b) using the given values.

_____

    d. Repeat parts (a–c) using centimeters instead of millimeters.

_____

6. Simplify.

    a. $\dfrac{(xy)^3}{xy^4}$

    b. $(3mn^5)^3$

_____   _____

    c. $(a^2b^{-3})(a^{-6}b^2)$

    d. $\left(\dfrac{cd^{-1}}{c^2d^4}\right)^{-2}$

_____   _____

7. Use the Pythagorean Theorem to label the missing lengths for these right triangles.

    a.

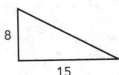

8
15

    b.

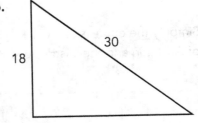

30
18

6-16 Writing Equivalent Expressions

Extra Practice

Use the Distributive Property to write the additive inverse of each of these expressions. Show your work. Simplify the expressions if necessary so that each expression shows the terms and coefficients as clearly as possible. Use brackets when needed.

1. $x + 1$

2. $-x + 1$

_____   _____

Sample

$a + 5$

The additive inverse is $-(a + 5) = -a - 5$.

3. $-(x + 1)$

4. $-(-x + 1)$

_____   _____

Sample

$-2(4a^3 + 6)$

The additive inverse is $-[-2(4a^3 + 6)] = 2(4a^3 + 6) = 8a^3 + 12$.

5. $x - 1$

6. $-(x - 1)$

_____   _____

7. $x - y$

8. $2x - 2y$

_____   _____

9. $-2x + 4y$

10. $x^5 - y^5$

_____   _____

Extra Practice continued _____

Use the Distributive Property to write the additive inverse of each of these expressions. Show your work. Simplify the expressions if necessary so that each expression shows the terms and coefficients as clearly as possible. Use brackets if they help you.

11. $-2x^5 - y^5$

_____

_____

12. $2x(x - y)$

_____

_____

13. $x + y + z$

_____

14. $-x + y - z$

_____

15. $\dfrac{x^2 + x}{x}$

_____

_____

16. $\dfrac{x^3 + x^2}{x^2}$

_____

_____

17. $-2x^4(x - 2y)$

_____

_____

18. $2xy(x^5 - y^5)$

_____

_____

19. $18\left(\dfrac{2}{3}x + \dfrac{1}{3}\right)$

_____

_____

_____

20. $-2x(x^2 - 4x + 6)$

_____

_____

_____

21. $\dfrac{7xy^2 - 3x^3y}{xy} \cdot \dfrac{1}{5}$

_____

_____

_____

22. $\dfrac{-6x^5 + 4x^3}{10x^3} \cdot 15$

_____

_____

_____

6-17 Using Expressions in Geometry

Extra Practice

1. Sketch area models to represent these expressions.

  a. $x(x + 2)$

                                        b. $5(x - 1)$

  c. $x(x + 2) - 5(x - 1)$

2. Explain your approach for constructing an area model for Problem 1(c).

_____

_____

_____

_____

3. Determine an alternate approach for constructing an area model for Problem 1(c). Explain the approach in words, and then sketch the alternative model.

_____

_____

_____

_____

_____

Extra Practice continued

4. Use the Distributive Property to write an expression equivalent to $5m + 5n + 10$.

_____

5. Sketch a geometric figure with an area that can be represented by either expression in Problem 4.

6. Think about these two expressions.

$x^2 + 9$ $\qquad\qquad\qquad\qquad$ $(x + 3)^2$

   a. Write verbal instructions for each of these expressions.

   _____

   _____

   b. Sketch an area model to represent each expression.

   c. Are these two expressions equivalent? Evaluate each expression for $x = 0$, $x = 1$, and $x = 2$, and explain how the results support your answer.

   _____

   _____

   _____

   _____

   _____

   _____

6-18 Writing Equations

Extra Practice

1. Identify which number property tells you the equation is a true statement.

   a. $5x + 10 + 15z = 5(x + 2 + 3z)$

   _____

   b. $(x - y)\frac{1}{2} = \frac{1}{2}(x - y)$

   _____

   c. $(2x)(yz) = 2(xyz)$

   _____

   d. $\frac{x}{2} + \frac{y}{10} = \frac{x}{2} \cdot \frac{5}{5} + \frac{y}{10}$

   _____

2. Jamal's grandfather is 85 years old. You know that last year Jamal's grandfather was 6 times older than Jamal. Write an equation that will help determine Jamal's age.

   _____

3. A rectangle is 8 feet long and 6 feet wide. If each dimension is increased by the same number of feet, the area of the new rectangle is 80 square feet. Write an equation for the new rectangle with x representing the increase in feet.

   _____

4. The height of a rectangle is 5 inches less than the length of its base, and the area of the rectangle is 52 square inches. Write an equation that will help determine the height of the rectangle.

   _____

   _____

Name _____ Class _____ Date _____

Extra Practice continued

5. The graph of the equation
$y = 2x + 8$ is shown at the right.

a. Identify the coordinates of at least one point on the line.

_____

b. Show that the coordinates of the point you identified in part (a) give a solution to the equation by substituting the x- and y-values into the equation and confirming that the equation is true.

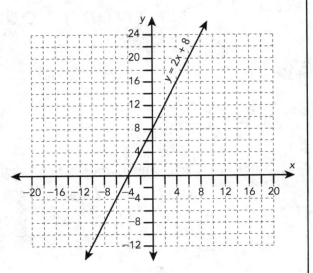

_____

c. Show that the point $(2, 8)$ is not a solution to the equation $y = 2x + 8$.

_____

6. The graph of the equation
$y = -3x - 3$ is shown at the right.

a. Identify the coordinates of at least one point on the line.

_____

b. Show that the coordinates of the point you identified in part (a) give a solution to the equation by substituting the x- and y-values into the equation and confirming that the equation is true.

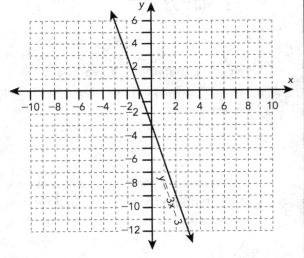

_____

c. Show that the point $(-2.2, 3.6)$ is a solution to the equation $y = -3x - 3$ and a solution to the equation $y = 2x + 8$.

_____

_____

6-19 The Addition Property of Equality

Extra Practice

1. This table shows examples that illustrate the Addition Property of Equality, with a, b, and c as numbers, variables, and expressions. Complete the table.

Beginning Equation		Change		Apply Property of Equality		Simplify to Write New Equation
$a = b$	**a.**			$a + c = b + c$		$a + c = b + c$
$z = x - 5$		add 5	**b.**			$z + 5 = x$
$7 + b = 12$	**c.**			$7 + b + (-7) = 12 + (-7)$		$b = 5$
d.		add -10		$x + 10 + (-10) = 0 + (-10)$		$x = -10$
$0.4 + y = 2.4$		add -0.4	**e.**			$y = 2$
$x - 2y = 25$		add $2y$	**f.**			$x = 25 + 2y$
g.		add $-4x$		$y + 4x + (-4x) = 4x + (-4x)$		$y = 0$
$4x + 6 = -10y$		add $10y$		$4x + 6 + 10y = -10y + 10y$	**h.**	
$4.5x - y = 0$		add y	**i.**			$4.5x = y$
$-\frac{1}{3}x + \frac{16}{3} = \frac{8}{3}x$		add $\frac{1}{3}x$		$-\frac{1}{3}x + \frac{16}{3} + \frac{1}{3}x = \frac{8}{3}x + \frac{1}{3}x$	**j.**	

Extra Practice continued

2. Lisa started with the equation $y = x + 1$.

a. She used one of the number properties to get the equation $y + 4 = x + 5$. What did she do?

_____

b. Lisa then changed $y + 4 = x + 5$ to $y - 1 = x$. What did she do?

_____

c. (0, 1) and (7, 8) are part of the solution set for Lisa's equation $y - 1 = x$. Identify three more pairs of (x, y) that are part of the solution set for this equation.

_____

d. Is it possible to find a pair of values that would be true for $y + 4 = x + 5$ or $y - 1 = x$ but not for $y = x + 1$? Explain your answer.

_____

e. Suppose $y = 19$. Solve Lisa's equation, $y = x + 1$, for x.

_____

3. Solve the equation. Justify each step with either the Addition Property of Equality, a number property, or an operation. Then check your solution.

a. $y + 12 = 0$

_____

_____

_____

b. $9(x - 3) = 10x$

_____

_____

_____

_____

Name _____ Class _____ Date _____

6-20 The Multiplication Property of Equality

Extra Practice

1. This table shows examples that illustrate the Multiplication Property of Equality, with a, b, and c as numbers, variables, and expressions. Complete the table.

Beginning Equation	Change	Apply Property of Equality	Simplify to Write New Equation
$a = b$	**a.**	$ac = bc$	$ac = bc$
$7x = 49$	multiply by $\frac{1}{7}$	**b.**	$x = 7$
$64 = 8y$	**c.**	$\frac{1}{8} \cdot 64 = \frac{1}{8} \cdot 8y$	$8 = y$
d.	multiply by 12	$12\left(\frac{x}{12}\right) = 12 \cdot 12$	$x = 144$
$0.4x = 25$	**e.**	$\frac{1}{0.4} \cdot 0.4x = \frac{1}{0.4} \cdot 25$	$x = 62.5$
$25y = 100$	**f.**	**g.**	$y = 4$

2. One solution to the equation $2p - 6 = 12$ is shown below. Fill in the justifications for each step in the solution. Then check the solution.

$2p - 6 + 6 = 12 + 6$ _____

$2p = 18$ _____

$\frac{1}{2} \cdot 2p = \frac{1}{2} \cdot 18$ _____

$p = 9$ _____

Check: _____

Extra Practice continued

3. Solve each equation using the properties of equality and the number properties. Then check your solution.

a. $3(x - 4) = 12$

b. $2(m - 6) - m = 12$

c. $7x - 2(x - 5) = 20$

d. $2(x - 7) - 4(x - 20) = 2x + 10$

6-21 Combining the Properties of Equality

Extra Practice

1. Solve the equation. Justify each step using the properties of equality, a number property, or an operation. Then check your solution.

a. $2a - 7 = -9$

_____

_____

_____

_____

_____

b. $-15 = 21 + 3b$

_____

_____

_____

_____

_____

c. $20 - 2.5g = -20$

_____

_____

_____

_____

_____

Name _____ Class _____ Date _____

Extra Practice continued

2. The senior class is going on a field trip. Five equal groups of students fill five of the buses, while 26 students ride on the last bus. If 281 students are going on the field trip, how many students are on each of the buses that are full? Write an equation that represents this situation. Then solve the equation, justifying each step with a property of equality, a number property, or an operation.

_____

_____

_____

_____

_____

3. Four friends buy tickets to a musical. After the show, the group spends $17 on ice cream. If the friends spent $90 total for the evening, how much did each ticket to the musical cost? Write an equation that represents this situation. Then solve the equation, justifying each step with a property of equality, a number property, or an operation.

_____

_____

_____

_____

_____

4. Dwayne is solving the equation $6n + 12 = 42$. He states that he can solve the equation by first multiplying both sides of the equation by $\frac{1}{6}$. Is Dwayne correct? Explain your answer.

_____

_____

_____

_____

_____

6-22 Solving Equations Requiring Simplification

Extra Practice

1. Solve the equation. Justify each step using the properties of equality, a number property, or an operation. Then check your solution.

a. $-4(x + 5) = 16$

_____

_____

_____

_____

_____

b. $3(a - 7) - 2a = -16$

_____

_____

_____

_____

_____

_____

_____

c. $6n - 4(n + 5) = -8$

_____

_____

_____

_____

_____

_____

_____

Name _____ Class _____ Date _____

Extra Practice continued

2. Consider the shaded region of the diagram below, formed by removing a smaller rectangle from a larger rectangle.

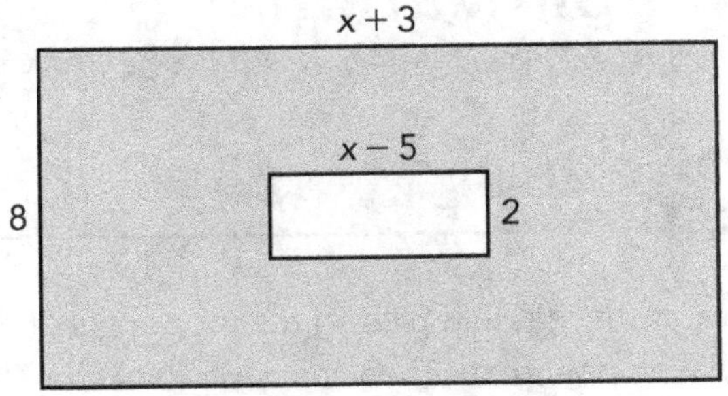

$x+3$

$x-5$

8   2

a. Write an expression for the area of the shaded region.

_____

b. Use your expression from part (a) to find x if the shaded area is 112 square units. Justify each step using the properties of equality, a number property, or an operation.

_____

_____

_____

_____

_____

_____

_____

c. What are the dimensions of the two rectangles in the figure?

_____

3. Lisa is solving the equation $-2(x+7)=10$. She states that she can solve the equation without using the Distributive Property. Is Lisa correct? Explain your answer.

_____

_____

_____

6-23 Inequalities

Extra Practice

1. Represent each situation with an inequality that includes a variable. For each situation, write three numbers that solve the inequality.

   a. To ride the roller coaster, your height must be at least 54 inches.

   _____

   b. Jamal's pulse was more than 10 beats per minute faster after he exercised.

   _____

   c. You can spend at most $8 on a movie and popcorn.

   _____

   d. To run for sheriff, you must be more than 30 years old.

   _____

   e. To get the senior citizen discount, your age must be at least 65.

   _____

   f. At the temperature of 32° or below, water freezes.

   _____

2. Describe the types of numbers (integers, decimals, negative, etc.) that fit each situation.

   a. To ride the roller coaster, your height must be at least 54 inches.

   _____

   _____

   b. Jamal's pulse was more than 10 beats per minute faster after he exercised.

   _____

   _____

   _____

   _____

Extra Practice continued

c. You can spend at most $8 on a movie and popcorn.

_____

_____

d. To run for sheriff, you must be more than 30 years old.

_____

_____

_____

e. To get the senior citizen discount, your age must be at least 65.

_____

_____

_____

f. At the temperature of 32° or below, water freezes.

_____

_____

_____

3. a. Think about the inequality $n + 7 > 15$. Is the solution $n > 8$? Say why or why not.

_____

_____

_____

b. Think about the inequality $45 < 3 + y$. Is the solution $y > 42$? Say why or why not.

_____

_____

_____

c. Think about the inequality $27 > t + 9$. Is the solution $t > 18$? Say why or why not.

_____

_____

_____

6-24 The Unit in Review

◼ Extra Practice

1. A person drives m miles towards a store that is 21 miles from her house. Write an expression for the number of miles the person still needs to drive to reach the store. _____

2. The price of hardcover books at a used book sale is $1.25 and the price of paperback books at the book sale is $0.40. It costs $2.00 to enter the book sale, and you get a 10-cent discount for bringing your own bag to carry the books home. Write an expression for the cost of h hardcover and p paperback books if you bring your own bag. Express your answer in both cents and in dollars.

_____

3. Describe a quantity that can be represented by the given expression.

   a. $8m$ _____

   b. $2n - 7$ _____

   _____

4. Evaluate the expression $4s - 9t + 11$ for $s = -2$ and $t = 3$. _____

5. a. Write a variable expression for these instructions.

   "Square a number, then multiply the result by 3, then add 5 times the number, and then add 7." _____

   b. Sketch an area model to represent the quantity described in part (a).

Extra Practice continued

6. Simplify.

  a. $(x^3y^4)(xy^3)^{-2}$ _____

  b. $\dfrac{(x^6y^8)^3}{x^3y}$ _____

7. Use the Pythagorean Theorem to determine whether or not the set of values {11, 60, 61} could be the sides of a right triangle. Explain why or why not.

_____

_____

8. Use the properties of equality and other number properties to solve $4x - 15 = 19$. Justify each step with a property or operation.

_____

_____

_____

_____

9. Show that each of the following (x, y) pairs is a solution to the linear equation: $\frac{3}{4}y = \frac{1}{8}x + \frac{1}{2}$.

  a. (2, 1) _____

  b. (8, 2) _____

  c. (−10, −1) _____

10. Solve the linear equation $y = -3x + 10$ for the corresponding x- or y-value given.

  a. Solve for x when $y = 4$. _____

  b. Solve for y when $x = -5$. _____

11. For each inequality, give three values for x that make the inequality true and three values for x that make the inequality false. Include a negative number and a number that is not an integer. Then represent the solution on a number line.

  a. $x - 3 > -4$ _____

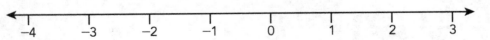

  b. $x - 3 \le -4$ _____

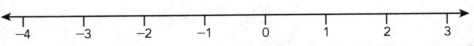